AF845468

QUALITY ASSURANCE IN BLOOD BANKING AND ITS CLINICAL IMPACT

DEVELOPMENTS IN HEMATOLOGY AND IMMUNOLOGY

Already published in this series:

Lijnen, H.R., Collen, D. and Verstraete, M., eds: Synthetic Substrates in Clinical Blood Coagulation Assays. 1980. ISBN 90-247-2409-0

Smit Sibinga, C.Th., Das, P.C. and Forfar, J.O., eds: Paediatrics and Blood Transfusion. 1982. ISBN 90-247-2619-0

Fabris, N., ed: Immunology and Ageing. 1982. ISBN 90-247-2640-9

Hornstra, G.: Dietary Fats, Prostanoids and Arterial Thrombosis. 1982. ISBN 90-247-2667-0

Smit Sibinga, C.Th., Das, P.C. and Loghem, van J.J., eds: Blood Transfusion and Problems of Bleeding. 1982. ISBN 90-247-3058-9

Dormandy, J., ed: Red Cell Deformability and Filterability. 1983. ISBN 0-89838-578-4

Quality Assurance in Blood Banking and Its Clinical Impact

Proceedings of the Seventh Annual Symposium on Blood Transfusion, Groningen 1982, organized by the Red Cross Blood Bank Groningen-Drenthe

edited by

C Th Smit Sibinga, P C Das
Red Cross Blood Bank Groningen-Drenthe, The Netherlands
H F Taswell
Mayo Clinic Blood Bank, Rochester MN, USA

1984 **MARTINUS NIJHOFF PUBLISHERS**
a member of the KLUWER ACADEMIC PUBLISHERS GROUP
BOSTON / THE HAGUE / DORDRECHT / LANCASTER

Distributors

for the United States and Canada: Kluwer Boston, Inc., 190 Old Derby Street, Hingham, MA 02043, USA
for all other countries: Kluwer Academic Publishers Group, Distribution Center, P.O.Box 322, 3300 AH Dordrecht, The Netherlands

Library of Congress Cataloging in Publication Data

Symposium on Blood Transfusion (7th : 1982 :
Groningen, Netherlands)
Quality assurance in blood banking and its clinical impact.

(Developments in hematology and immunology)
1. Blood-banks--Quality control--Congresses. 2. Blood --Transfusion--Safety measures--Congresses. I. Smit Sibinga, C. Th. II. Das, P. C. III. Taswell, Howard F. IV. Stichting Rode Kruis Bloedbank Groningen/Drente. V. Title. VI. Series.
RM172.S96 1982 362.1'784 83-23665
ISBN 0-89838-618-7

ISBN 0-89838-618-7 (this volume)
ISBN 90-247-2432-5 (series)

Copyright

© 1984 by Martinus Nijhoff Publishers, Boston.

All rights reserved. No part of this publication may be reproduced, stored in a retrieval system, or transmitted in any form or by any means, mechanical, photocopying, recording, or otherwise, without the prior written permission of the publishers,
Martinus Nijhoff Publishers, 190 Old Derby Street, Hingham, MA 02043, USA.

PRINTED IN THE NETHERLANDS

TRAVENOL

Acknowledgement

This publication has been made possible through the support of Travenol, which is gratefully acknowledged.

CONTENTS

INVITED SPEAKERS

J-P. Allain	- Centre National de Transfusion Sanguine, Paris, France
H. de Beus	- Wilhelmina Hospital, Assen, The Netherlands
F. Bonanni	- Travenol International Services Inc., Brussels, Belgium
A.F. Casparie	- Weezenlanden Hospital, Zwolle, The Netherlands
M. Clay	- American Red Cross Blood Services, St. Paul, MN, USA
R.J. Crawford	- Glascow and West of Scotland Blood Transfusion Service, Glasgow, UK
P.C. Das (moderator)	- Red Cross Blood Bank Groningen-Drenthe, Groningen, The Netherlands
J.A. van der Does (moderator)	- Red Cross Blood Bank 's Gravenhage, The Netherlands
J.W. Dorpema (moderator)	- State Control Laboratory, National Institute of Health, Bilthoven, The Netherlands
M.R. Halie (moderator)	- Dept. of International Medicine, University of Groningen, Groningen, The Netherlands
A.M. Holburn (on behalf of WHO)	- Blood Group Reference Laboratory, Oxford, UK
S.R. Holan	- National Institute of Haematology and Blood Transfusion, Budapest, Hungary
R.E. Klein (moderator)	- National Committee on I & A, AABB, Arlington, VA, USA
J. Leikola	- League of Red Cross Societies, Geneva, Switzerland
W.L. Marsh	- The New York Blood Center, New York, NY, USA

H. van der Meulen	- University of Groningen, Groningen, The Netherlands
B.A. Myhre (moderator)	- University of California, Los Angeles, CA, USA
H.W. Reesink	- Amsterdam Medical Centre, Amsterdam, The Netherlands
Ch.A. Shiffer (moderator)	- University of Maryland Cancer Center, Baltimore, MD, USA
P.J. Schmidt	- Southwest Florida Blood Bank, Tampa, FL, USA
K. Sintnicolaas	- Daniël den Hoed Clinic, Rotterdam, The Netherlands
Z. Smit	- Red Cross Blood Bank Groningen-Drenthe, Groningen, The Netherlands
C.Th. Smit Sibinga (moderator)	- Red Cross Blood Bank Groningen-Drenthe, Groningen, The Netherlands
Ch.L. Sonnenberg (moderator)	- Mayo Clinic Blood Bank, Rochester, MN, USA
H.F. Taswell (chairman)	- Mayo Clinic Blood Bank, Rochester, MN, USA

FOREWORD
THE PHILOSOPHY OF QUALITY ASSURANCE IN THE BLOOD BANK

H.F. Taswell

One year before this symposium, Cees Smit Sibinga and I began to discuss an approach to quality assurance in the blood bank which we felt would be both important and practical and could serve as the basis for the choice of subjects to be presented in the symposium. As an introduction to this book, I would like to outline our approach, the subjects chosen and the rationale behind our choice.

What is the fundamental purpose of a blood bank and transfusion service? Simply stated, the purpose of a blood bank and transfusion service and of a quality assurance program in blood banking is, for the one to provide and, the other to assure safe and effective transfusion therapy. This objective is in contrast to that of other clinical laboratories. The objective in a clinical chemistry laboratory is to produce accurate test results which will be meaningful to the clinician taking care of his patient. In most clinical laboratories, therefore, the goals of a quality assurance program are largely quantitative, that is, to assure accurate numerical test results. In contrast, in the blood bank, the goals of quality assurance are primarily qualitative, that is, to assure safe and effective transfusion. As a result, two somewhat different approaches to quality assurance are necessary.

How are we to assure quality in the blood bank? Safe and effective transfusion can be achieved to a large degree by prevention of error. Blood bank procedures are repetitive and relatively simple and straight forward. Since the morbidity and mortality associated with transfusion arises primarily from errors, one of the primary goals of quality assurance in the blood bank should be the prevention of errors.

What is an error? An error can be defined for the purpose of this introduction as an "inadvertent or unauthorized deviation from standard procedure". If one accepts that errors are the primary cause of transfusion morbidity and mortality and that an error is a deviation from standard procedure, then the necessary elements of a quality assurance program in the blood bank are readily apparent. These same elements will provide both a means of error control and an efficient management system.

What are the necessary elements? The first and most important element needed for a quality assurance program is a standardized written procedure for every test and every service which that blood bank and/or transfusion service intends to provide to donors, patients and physicians. These procedures must be based on generally accepted goals or standards.

Once the standard procedure has been written, who will implement it? Different procedures entail different kinds of tasks and require different kinds of people. Therefore, it is necessary to define the responsibilities and personnel needs required to fulfill each procedure. Separate job descriptions must be written for each employee group with responsibility for a different type of procedure. Although the job description is generally thought of as a management tool, it is, in fact, just as much a tool of quality assurance. A well-written job description will permit evaluation of competency for the position and aid in the selection of the most appropriate individual from those who are available. Once personnel are selected, awareness of their duties permits development of appropriate initial training, continuing education and performance appraisal.

More traditional, but, of course, equally important are quality assurance of equipment and reagents. The user and manufacturer each must take somewhat different approaches to quality assurance of equipment or reagents. For the user, the approach to quality assurance of equipment and reagents is, in many respects, similar to that for personnel.

What is a particular reagent or piece of equipment expected to do? As with personnel, it is necessary to first define the task to be performed by equipment or by reagents; i.e., to develop "a job description". Knowing the task to be achieved, it is then necessary to select from among the wide variety of equipment or reagents available. Once selected, it is necessary to establish a maintenance program to assure that equipment or reagents continue to perform as expected. Maintenance of reagents, although quite different from maintenance of equipment, is equally important and requires proper labeling, handling and storage, if they are to perform as intended.

How well is the blood bank fulfilling its purpose? To assure that the expected performance of reagents, equipment, personnel or their products is, in fact, achieved, a most important element of a quality assurance program is the monitoring of performance. Theoretically, if we have selected appropriate procedures and suitable personnel, equipment and reagents, we should obtain accurate results and safe and effective products and services. Obviously, this does not always happen. Therefore, it is important to evaluate each of the end products of a blood bank or transfusion service. One type of evaluation is through proficiency testing which can be done either with periodic proficiency test materials provided by external sources, i.e., various national and international agencies, or on a more continuous basis, by the use of proficiency samples devised by and distributed within the home laboratory. Since the products of the blood bank and transfusion service are quite varied and may be either a test result, some type of service or a blood product such as a unit of blood or platelets, their evaluation cannot always be attained through proficiency testing alone. Evaluation of blood products for their safety and effectiveness is achieved by other techniques, usually a combination of in vitro and in vivo product testing.

A third approach to evaluation of the blood bank's products and services is through the recognition and analysis of errors. Because of the significant association between blood bank errors and transfusion morbidity and mortality, error recognition, analysis and control is a most important (and previously neglected) aspect of quality assurance. There are two fundamental methods of quality assurance utilizing error analysis to evaluate the products of the blood bank. One method is through the use of intentional errors which are placed periodically throughout the blood bank. The primary purpose of this method is to provide blood bank management and employees with an estimate of their ability to detect errors. Their observed ability to detect intentional errors, in turn provides a measure of their ability to detect unintentional (or real) errors. The second part of an error analysis program requires the recognition, description and recording of all errors. If all errors are recognized and reported in a consistent manner, it becomes possible to determine the frequency of unintentional errors (as modified by our knowledge of the detection rate of intentional errors), the type of errors, where they are occurring, what is causing them and how they can be corrected.

The following chapters discuss in more detail the fundamentals of quality control in blood banking as they relate to principles, standards, procedures, personnel, equipment, reagents, clinical efficacy, and error analysis and as they aid in achieving safe and effective transfusion.

OPENING ADDRESS

A.M. Holburn

First I would like to present the apologies of Dr. F. Lothe of the Division of Health Laboratory Technology of the WHO in Geneva. He was unfortunately not able to come. I stand in his place and I am very pleased to be able to represent the WHO in making these opening remarks.

The WHO is very conscious of the vital role that laboratories play in patient care. There are roughly 65,000 clinical laboratories in the WHO European Region alone and in most the workload has increased enormously in recent years.

One aspect of Quality Assurance to which the WHO has addressed itself in some detail is that of External Quality Assessment (EQA). EQA is a system of objectively checking laboratory results by means of an external agency. Analysis of results involves a comparison of individual laboratories' results with those of all other laboratories. The main object is to establish between laboratory compatibility. In 1979 the WHO invited a number of experts to pool the experiences gained from their national EQA schemes. The group was asked to consider the need for EQA schemes, to consider the respective roles that should be played by governments and scientists, to consider their design and also the benefits that could be obtained from such schemes. The group was further asked to make recommendations that could be helpful in countries in which the development of Quality Assessment Schemes has been slow or non existent.

The first crucial question is who should carry the main responsibility for external assessment of clinical laboratories. Should they be government agencies or the relevant professional societies? The Working Group concluded that governments have the prime responsibility for establishing official EQA schemes for clinical laboratories and that this may be seen as one part of their overall responsibility for ensuring adequate standards of health care. The group was, however, equally clear in its conclusion that scientists and not administrators should design, organise and operate the schemes. The chosen scientists must have wide and recent experience of the laboratory practices that they are attempting to monitor. In virtually all European countries which have established EQA the schemes do in fact operate through some kind of co-operation between government and groups of professional scientists. Governments have established official schemes, ensured that they are adequately funded and in some countries have also introduced legislation to oblige laboratories to participate. Most national EQA schemes originated in unofficial schemes launched by individual scientists with a particular interest in this work. With increasing governmental involvement these schemes have developed into large scale schemes monitoring an ever widening range of laboratory acitivities. Quality Assessment is, therefore, itself one of the rapid growth areas of laboratory medicine. Eventually the value of individual schemes will have to be proven in order to justify the resources employed in them.

Participation in EQA schemes can be either voluntary or obligatory. On the principle that one volunteer is worth two conscripts the former might appear to be the better course. A volunteer is more likely to enter into the spirit of the schemes. The schemes are, or should be, essentially educational. The organisers and participants should share a desire to improve standards and participants should not fear that weaker laboratories will be hounded unceremoniously out of business. Unfortunately, it is in the nature of things that not everyone who should volunteer does so. Fortunately, various means are at hand which may be used to facilitate participation in voluntary schemes. One is simply to make the scheme free to participants. Another, and rather more effective way is for professional bodies to withdraw approval for training of any laboratory that will not participate. Governmental intervention in the form of legislation is not, therefore, essential to the running of these schemes although governmental interest in the form of financing the schemes is very much to be desired.

Probably the best time to encourage voluntary participation is when a scheme is in process of being established. It may take a bit of time to get a new scheme running satisfactorily. There are many teething problems to be overcome and it does not seem reasonable to compel participation in an untried scheme. In a well run voluntary scheme confidence will gradually develop between the participants and the organisers. In order to achieve such confidence the organisers must be open to and responsive to scientific criticism. They must also be able to justify the scientific basis and mode of operation of their schemes and they must be prepared to do so in open meetings.

After a scheme has run successfully for several years and confidence in the scientific validity of the scheme has been established then a different approach to participation may be justified. At this stage professional societies can reasonably insist that all laboratories participate. Central government, which may be funding the scheme also has a legitimate interest. Governments cannot be expected to continue to finance schemes if an unknown proportion of laboratories choose not to participate, or if some laboratories simply discontinue participation if their results are poor and if they do not seek assistance to remedy their deficiencies.

There appears to be ample scope for international co-operation in EQA even between countries with highly developed schemes. The prime purpose of EQA is to establish inter-laboratory comparability. In the various national schemes in blood group serology which have been developed so far, there are considerable differences in the design of the exercises, in the nature of the test materials issued and in the expression of results. These differences make it difficult or impossible to compare standards of performance between countries and ultimately we shall want to now if differences in national practices are associated with differences in performance. Organisers of new schemes should therefore avoid designing highly individual schemes which will not permit information obtained within national borders to be interpreted in the light of results obtained elsewhere. The WHO did not, however, recommend expansion of existing national schemes into international schemes. The reason for this was only in part the administrative difficulties. A more important reason for not expanding is that the educational function of EQA is most readily undertaken on a local basis. It is the national groups of scientists who are best placed to come to the assistance of weaker laboratories. Indeed the organisers of the schemes are frequently able to offer quick and informal advice to individual participants. There is little purpose in operating expensive schemes if participants cannot obtain ready access to help and advice. As much effort should go into providing this supportive role as into the scheme itself. In this way the interests of patients will best be served.

Finally I would like to wish you a most interesting and enjoyable meeting. Thank you.

I. Principles and organization of quality assurance

INTERNATIONAL ORGANIZATION OF QUALITY ASSURANCE

J. Leikola

The blood programmes in different countries may be organized by government or other public agencies, by the Red Cross or by private enterprises. In a recent survey of 32 countries, done for the ISH/ISBT Congress in Budapest in 1982, Professor S.R. Hollán found that, in 14 countries there was a governmental blood programme, in 11 countries, the blood services were organized exclusively by Red Cross whilst only one country was entirely dependent on private bloodbanks. In the remaining five countries, there were different types of services.

There are three worldwide international organizations that are dealing with questions related to bloodtransfusion: World Health Organization (WHO), International Society of Bloodtransfusion (ISBT) and League of Red Cross Societies (LRCS). At the WHO headquarters, the matters are handled by the Division of Diagnostic, Therapeutic and Rehabilitative Technology, particulary by its Biologicals Unit and Health Laboratory Technology Unit. The League of Red Cross Societies has a Bloodtransfusion Service as an administrative unit.

These three international organizations have emphasized the need for quality assurance in every bloodtransfusion service, whether a small blood bank with just basic functions or a large centre with fractionation facilities. WHO and LRCS published jointly in 1971 a Guide to the Formation and operation of a transfusion service (1,2). The concept of quality control was at that time not as readily connected with bloodtransfusion activities as it is today, but the need to set standards and to follow the quality of products and procedures was clearly indicated.

WHO recently published a document entitled: "The collection, fractionation, quality control and uses of blood and blood products" (3). This book deals with plasmapheresis, albumin solutions, coagulation factors and immunoglobulin preparations. Guidelines are given on the quality control of albumin solutions and of Factor VIII. The document makes rather general statements about quality assurance and leaves it to the individual countries and centres to design detailed procedures to assure the quality of plasma derivatives. Reference is made to the requirements for the control of plasma fractions, which were originally drawn up in 1978 by a team of WHO consultants and staff members and approved by the

WHO Expert Committee on Biological Standardization (4). All the requirements for collection, processing and quality control of human blood and blood products are given as an annex to the WHO document.

ISBT has published booklets on different aspects of bloodtransfusion. The Guid Number 3 is devoted to quality assurance in the bloodtransfusion service (5). This guide, originally drafted by B.A. Myhre, emphasizes the need to have quality assurance procedures at every step of blood donation, processing and transfusion. As stated in the Guide, there are two major requirements for the proper operation of a bloodtransfusion laboratory: firstly, that the test results should be accurate, meaningful and unchallengeable; secondly, that the products prepared should contain an adequate concentration of the stated component(s) and minimal concentrations of unwanted components. Since its publication in 1978, the Guide has proved very useful for many blood centres. Not only does it adopt a practical approach, but it also gives new impetus to the idea of having an organized way to assure the final quality of the products.

In European conditions, except for plasma fractionation, there are few national regulations on organization of quality control in bloodtransfusion services. The increasing importance of this aspect has been recognized by the Council of Europe and it has established a select committee of experts to deal with automation and quality control in bloodtransfusion services. The select committee has the task of preparing guidelines for quality control in blood banks covering especially those aspects of collecting and processing blood that are not included in the pharmacopoeias or in Good Manufacturing Procedures. The guidelines are expected to be ready in 1983. They contain criteria for selection of blood donors. There are recommendations for standards and arrangements of quality assurance procedures concerning blood collection, separation of blood components, storage, issue and transportation of blood as well as various laboratory procedures. Also included are instructions for quality control of transfusion practices, of equipment and record keeping.

Some other international organizations, in addition to the four mentioned above, sometimes touch on matters that are related to quality assurance in bloodtransfusion services. These are the International Organization for Standardization, the International Committee for Standardization in Haematology, the World Federation of Hemophilia and the International Federation of Blood Donor Organizations. Commercial organizations, e.g. International Federation of Pharmaceutical Manufacturers Associations, have a keen interest in the requirements of quality control in plasma fractionation. There is much trade of plasma between different countries and in order to assure the high quality of end products, establishment and implementation of quality control in the source country is of prime importance.

Some national quality assurance programmes also have members from abroad. A few European centres participate regularly in the proficiency testing programmes of American organizations. Likewise, some of the leading centres act as reference laboratories for organized quality control in foreign countries. This activity is to be encouraged since it greatly facilitates the standardization of quality assurance on a practical level.

An exchange of blood samples has been very useful in proficiency testing and comparison of methods as applied in different countries. For several years, such an exchange has existed between centres that are represented in the above mentioned Select Committee of Experts of the Council of Europe. When serum samples containing unknown amounts of anti-D were distributed to several European countries over a considerable period of time, a remarkable improvement in the homogeneity of the results was achieved (6). The same was noted for HBsAg and anti-HBs.

Internationally, there seems to be an increasing interest in the field of quality assurance of bloodtransfusion services. It is important that views and experiences are exchanged across the borders. All the measures are aimed at safeguarding the quality of blood and blood products for transfusion. The most important duty of any transfusion service is to make it reasonably sure that blood donation is safe for the donor and that the recipient of blood is not challenged with unnecessary risks in connection with hemotherapy.

REFERENCES

1. Bowley, C.C., Goldsmith, K.L.G., Maycock, W.d'A., eds. Bloodtransfusion. A Guide to the formation and operation of a bloodtransfusion service. World Health Organization, Geneva 1971.
2. Cazal, P., Maycock, W.d'A. Addendum 1978. Bloodtransfusion. A Guide to the formation and operation of a bloodtransfusion service. World Health Organization, Geneva 1978.
3. World Health Organization. The collection, fractionation, quality control, and uses of blood and blood products. WHO, Geneva 1981.
4. WHO Expert Committee on Biological Standardization. Requirements for the collection, processing and quality control of human blood and blood products. WHO Technical Report Series No. 626, Annex 1, 1978:28–93.
5. ISBT Guid 3. Quality assurance in the bloodtransfusion laboratory. International Society of Bloodtransfusion, Paris 1978.
6. Moore, B.P.L., Wagstaff, W. Autoanalyzer quantification of anti-D: Results of an international proficiency survey. Rev. Fr. Transf. Immuno-Hématologie 1980;23:319–26.

A NATIONAL FRAMEWORK OF BLOOD TRANSFUSION ORGANIZATION

J.W. Dorpema

1. QUALITY CONTROL AND QUALITY ASSURANCE

Quality assurance, and more generally the interest to regard industrial and social processes as object of quality, has increased extremely over the past decade. It is very appropriate on this moment, in this country and on this spot to go into more detail on what the nestor of quality control, Dr. Duran, recently expressed as "life behind the dykes of quality control" (1). To continue this metaphor we could say that the industrialized countries have built quality dykes, in order to assure that products will function properly.

We should be aware of the fact that thinking in terms of quality is an attitude that has to be teached and has to be learned before it can function in an effective way. If this has been achieved than – according to Williamson – two methods are available to execute quality control. He distinguishes between (a) inductive and (b) deductive methods (2). The inductive methods are primarily oriented towards a preventive approach. This is because they are based on the application of criteria developed for the structure, the process and its results. In deductive methods the unsatisfactory results are the points of initiation of quality control. An analysis of the process leading to it must elucidate the causes of this unwanted and unexpected results. So this last approach must be defined as acting curative instead of preventive.

The industrial developments in the past two decades have shown that the quality thinking has evoluted tremendously and is still speeding up. So it is quite feasible that Dr. Feigenbaum, a US professor in quality control, stated at a recent European symposium on this subject: "Quality for future life will be a crucial theme" (3). That this statement is correct, can be illustrated by the example of the automobile industry. In order to raise the poor quality of the Japanese cars the concept of quality control circles was induced and optimalized in the early sixties. It is well known how successful this decision turned out to be.

In this context the fact that quality control circles must be marked as a system should be stressed, where the quality thinking has been incorporated largely in the production process (Figure 1). As a consequence quality control shifts more and more to quality

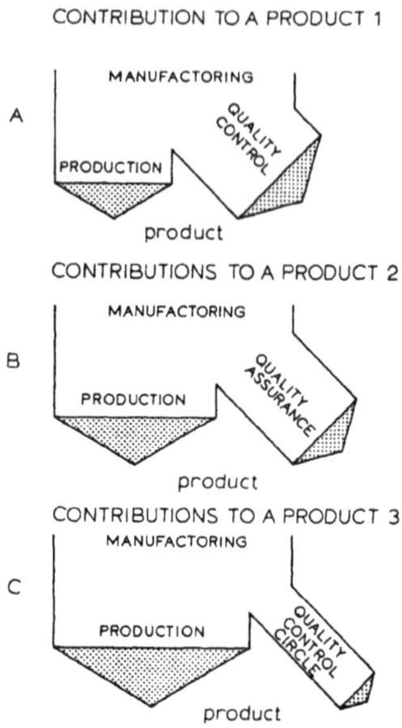

Figure 1

assurance. The monitoring function is reduced. Education, instruction and process-programming have become the main targets of the quality department. At this moment quality control circles is the hot topic in the US and Europe. Recently British Leyland has incorporated this system in the production of their Jaguar automobiles. As a result they could withdraw their inspectors. Lately in the Netherlands a stimulation arrangement called "Innovative Management 1982" has introduced the possibility to support small businesses financially, if they intend to introduce quality systems. So, the Japanese automobile industry has provided a real start for the incorporation of quality thinking in manufacturing processes.

Another conclusion which can be made from this is that the thinking in terms of quality has already spread widely. Hence we could say that quality will become a mentality. Moreover it implies that a society only can execute quality control when focusing both on the technical and social improvements.

2. QUALITY AND BLOODTRANSFUSION

What are the pathways to apply and promote quality in a special discipline as bloodtransfusion is supposed to be?

First of all a framework will be needed, a framework which is constructed by the general requirements for a national quality control system. These requirements are:

a. a general quality awareness must be created;
b. expertise in this field must be built up;
c. a structurized national quality policy must be established;
d. these efforts must result in an international approval of this policy.

3. BLOODTRANSFUSION IN THE NETHERLANDS

Now, what kind of picture would we get if we parachute these requirements on bloodtransfusion in The Netherlands, and relate this to the comments made about quality thinking.

The way bloodtransfusion is organized in a country is, like a lot of other activities, depending on and to a certain extend a reflection of its social and political structure.

To start we have to look back into history. Over the past few years the Dutch bloodtransfusion organization has been confronted with some problems. This, in itself, is not rather unique. Many organizations and institutions nowadays are not able to keep up with rapidly changing conditions. Of course, these events are extra stressed in times of socio-economical depression. An analysis of the situation showed that at one hand the legislation was not any more in compliance with the present circumstances, while, at the other hand, the bloodtransfusion system developed from bloodtransfusion services to blood banks, which resulted into a rather dispers field of activities. From this it can be concluded that such a situation is not a good climate for quality awareness. Controlling circuits and elements will not be able to function optimally. So it can be predicted that sooner or later such a system will be offended. For the Dutch bloodtransfusion organization where being self-supporting is one of the basic principles, the permission to import Factor VIII concentrate can be considered as an example of such an offence.

One of the positive aspects of an economical depression is that it increases the willingness to renew and change. It leads to creative impulses by which positive changes are more readily achieved. Obviously the restructuring process of the Dutch bloodtransfusion system originated from such an impulse.

In this restructuring process two trails can be distinguished. At one hand a governmental working group prepared a new act, while at the other hand the Dutch National Red Cross Organization contracted the former Dutch Minister of Health and Environmental Health, Dr. Ginjaar, in order to present a proposal for the renovation of the structure of the national bloodtransfusion organization. It has to be emphasized that this double trail strategy did not affect the basic principles of the Dutch system, which are:

a. blood is a national resource;
b. the donation system is non-remunerated and based on a voluntary gift;

c. the system must be self-supporting;
d. the transfer of blood from donor to patient must be regulated by working standards;
e. there is a public accountability.

At present, both trails are to be interconnected. It will result in a situation where the responsibilities of both government and other parties involved, are clearly separated. The government will set the criteria for the bloodtransfusion organization to function. In terms of quality control this would mean that the government will use the inductive method. A summary of the significant elements of the proposed Act clearly illustrates this:

1. Bloodtransfusion will be coordinated by a board, which compiles all parties involved in it. This board will advise the government in legislative and control matters. The board is supported by expert committees.
2. The expertise in bloodbanking will be regulated by enactments.
3. Also by decree there will be requirements for the annual production and the allocation of blood banks.
4. Donors will be protected by requirements.
5. The collection, processing, packaging and distribution will be regulated.
6. Importation of blood products will be prohibited unless a proven need exists which cannot be fulfilled by a national product.
7. Exportation is centralized.

So there is a framework. Certainly some effort and time will be needed to get the system completely filled in. Consultations and cooperation between government and those involved in bloodtransfusion will be a condition to make the whole system effective.

Also the deductive approach can be traced in this new Act: governmental officials can be assigned to the meetings of the board.

4. IMPLEMENTATION OF QUALITY ASSURANCE IN DUTCH BLOODBANKING

Previously it was stipulated that elements of quality thinking are incorporated in the renewed structure of bloodtransfusion in The Netherlands. Moreover, quality aspects will be largely represented in the collection, processing, packaging and distribution of blood. However, there is one aspect of bloodtransfusion that is not regulated in this new structure and that is the clinical application.

Bloodtransfusion organization has a social and a technical responsibility. It is intended to transfer blood and blood products from donors to patients. Both for ethical and economical reasons this transfer must be accomplished as efficient as possible. Just like all medical-pharmaceutical products, also blood and blood products have to obey the basic product requirements. So, they must be (a) safe, (b) effective and (c) properly produced. The requirements for proper production and to a large extent for safety, can be controlled by Good Manufacturing Practice (GMP), Good Laboratory Practice (GLP), regulations and prescribed tests. However, to get a qualitative impression of efficacy, and especially the clinical efficacy, is much more complicated. If the clinical application is not regulated and standardized than all quality of the product can easily be disturbed or even destroyed. The government also has to face this problem. However, there are ways to overcome. In this respect, the relation between the Dutch National Institue of Healt (RIV) and a Dutch Hemophilia Clinic, the Van Creveld Clinic, can serve as an illustration, where the government becomes informed about the quality of f.i. Factor VIII concentrates. Or in terms of quality thinking, a deductive approach which will evolute into inductive. An inductive approach which transfers and extends GMP to become Good Hospital Practice (GHP).

In conclusion, Alvin Toffler, in his last bestseller "The third wave" predicts a biotechnical and electronical revolution, which consequently will have a number of social implications (4). Therefore he concludes that countries with a highly developed and flexible democracy like The Netherlands would be predisposed to fulfill a guide function in this process. It is my expectation that some of it could become reality for bloodtransfusion.

REFERENCES

1. Duran, J.J. Quality for future life. Proceedings of the Annual EOQC conference. Stichting Kwaliteitsdienst KDI, Rotterdam (The Netherlands) 1982.
2. Williamson, J.S. Assessing and Improving Health Care Outcomes: The health accounting approach. Cambridge, Massachusetts (US) 1978.
3. Feigenbaum, A.V. Quality for future life. Proceedings of the Annual EOQC conference. Stichting Kwaliteitsdienst KDI, Rotterdam (The Netherlandc) 1982.
4. Toffler, A. The Third Wave. Pan Books Ltd., London 1981.

BLOOD TRANSFUSION PRACTICE IN HOSPITALS: A TOPIC FOR QUALITY ASSURANCE

A.F. Casparie

INTRODUCTION

Quality assurance in bloodbanking is well established, and sophisticated methods are developed for this purpose. However, the evaluation of blood transfusion practice does not get the same attention. Therefore, it seems necessary to focus attention on the quality of bloodtransfusion practice inside the hospital. To achieve this, medical audit can be a suitable instrument.

Over the past years there has developed in The Netherlands a growing interest in structured activities designed to assure the quality of medical care in hospitals: i.e. medical audit or peer review. In many hospitals the medical staff has formed a medical audit committee that applies quality assurance as a problem-oriented activity, e.g. oriented towards the resolving of a real problem in medical care delivery. In this process six steps can be distinguished (Table I). After the choice of the subject to be studied is made, criteria are developed by the involved physicians. Next, the practice of the delivered care is measured; then, if necessary a change in medical care is introduced; final a re-assessment is carried out.

Table I. Subsequent steps in a quality assurance study.

Selection of a topic	Comparison of criteria versus data
Development of criteria	Introduction of a change
Gathering of data	Re-assessment

BLOODTRANSFUSION PRACTICE: A GOOD TOPIC?

One of the topics for quality assurance frequently mentioned by medical audit committees is the practice of bloodtransfusion. Indeed, bloodtransfusion therapy seems a suitable topic for quality assurance for several reasons (Table II). Moreover, the few studies which have been published in the last two decades do suggest that a high percentage of bloodtransfusions is unneces-

Table II. Reasons for choosing bloodtransfusion therapy as a topic for quality assurance.

Administration of blood is a frequently occurring therapy in hospitals.
Indications for the use of blood in anaemic for bleeding patients are not sharply defined.
Use of blood or blood components can involve short-term as well as long-term complications.
Administration of blood involves financial costs.
Donation of blood is voluntary, that implies a greater responsibility for those who establish the indication for transfusion.

Table III. Flow sheet for bloodtransfusion practice.

Physician	- establishes the (eventual) indication - determines the proper type of blood component (packed cells, filtrated or washed erythrocytes) - determines if the unit will be given immediately or set in the assigned state
Laboratory and/or Blood Bank	- determines blood group (and antibodies) of the patient - looks for a suitable donor - has selected the donor and takes blood from this donor - processes the blood into the requested component - carries out the cross-match - delivers the bag to the department
Department or operating room	- controls names and blood group on the bag with the information mentioned in the patient record - connects the bag to the patient - carries out the controls
Physician	- treats any (eventual) complications and reports them to the laboratory and Blood Bank

Table IV. Topics in quality assurance of bloodtransfusion practice.

Indications for transfusion	Supply management and outdating of blood
Components of blood to be used	Treatment and registration of complications

sary. In 1960, Graham-Stewart (1) found that, even when all the clinicians were aware of the survey, 6,5% of all units of blood was given unnecessarily. In 1964, Diethrich (2) assessed that in his hospital 25% of multiple transfusions was not indicated when compared with his own criteria. Friedman (3) reported in 1978 that in a random number of hospitals in the USA, many patients without serious anaemia (hemoglobin more than 6,2 mmol/l) receive a transfusion. Recently in a first survey in our hospital we have found that 23% of all administrated units of blood did not meet our own criteria for indication (4).

THE PROCEDURE OF THE QUALITY ASSURANCE STUDY

Once the topic of bloodtransfusion therapy has been chosen for study, the next step in the process of quality assurance is the development of criteria for optimal management. Therefore, first we must know how this practice is organized. To make this clear, a flow-sheet can be of help (Table III). The beginning of the procedure, lies with the physician establishing the indications for transfusion. All other activities in the blood bank, the laboratory, the clinical department or the operation room are derived from that action. When focussing further on the physician, four items can be distinguished, to which attention must be payed (Table IV). For these four items, the medical staff must develop guidelines and the practice must be monitored. It is evident that under-transfusion will not be measured.

THE INDICATIONS FOR THE TRANSFUSION

Assurance of the validity of the indication must be the central point in bloodtransfusion therapy. However, it is not easy to find clear guidelines for transfusion indications in the literature. Wintrobe warns about the deplorable practice of transfusing patients whenever their hemoglobin value is below an arbitrarily set figure (5). Furthermore, the clinical situation will vary from patient to patient and it is not possible to develop criteria for all circumstances. Nevertheless, in measuring the quality of transfusion practice, one needs some guidelines. Otherwise, the judgement of the quality will be very subjective and implicit.

In studies on transfusion practice some criteria have been used. Diethrich stated that in the preoperative patient a hemoglobin below 6,2 mmol/l represents a positive indication for bloodtransfusion. In patients with a chronic anaemia, a hemoglobin of 4,4 mmol/l was set by him as an indication if the patient is symptomatic. Mc Coy (6) used as indications: 6,2 mmol/l in the preoperative patient, 4,4 mmol/l in patients with chronic anaemia and 6,2 mmol/l when complicating factors such as cardiac insufficiency are present. Crosby (7) stated that for a sedentary life 6,2 mmol/l hemoglobin is often sufficient and that even most bed-ridden patients are comfortable with 4,0 mmol/l.

In a recent study in our hospital (4) we used differentiated criteria, e.g. in patients between 25 and 50 years with a post-operative or chronic anaemia, a hemoglobin of 6,0 mmol/l indicates transfusion, and if there are complicating factors such as angina pectoris, 6,5 mmol/l is the limit.

However, there has been no clinical study reported that had proved that these criteria are valid. Thus the afore mentioned criteria depend more on clinical experience and conviction then on scientific research. Therefore, in anaemic patients without overt bleeding each medical staff must develop their own criteria for transfusion indications. Most authors agree that in patients with acute blood loss as during operation, transfusion is indicated when loss is more than 20% of the circulating blood volume (8).

The administration of one pint of blood is often considered as a misuse and can serve as an indication of bad overall transfusion practice. In several studies (1,2,9,10,11,12) it has been reported that 40% to 80% of all single unit transfusions were not indicated. However, it is dangerous to abandon all single unit transfusions, because some physicians will give two instead of one to avoid criticism. Besides that, during operation the blood loss can turn out to be less than was expected and after one unit of blood, transfusion therapy will be ended rightly. Nevertheless, it is justified that in a quality assurance study all single unit blood-transfusions must be investigated for electivity.

As a rough indication for eventual overuse in bloodtransfusion the mean use of blood per patient in hospital can be measured. This number can be compared with other hospitals under comparable circumstances.

THE COMPONENT OF BLOOD TO BE USED

The literature contains several guidelines for selective use of the proper blood component. Based on these guidelines the hospital staff can set explicit criteria for good medical care. As indications for packed cells versus whole blood, Bear (13) stated that only in acute blood loss whole blood should be used but that in the anaemic patient, packed red cells should always be used. Furthermore, in the literature criteria are mentioned about the use of filtrated or washed erythrocytes. The best indications are in cases with transfusion reactions caused by the presence of leucocytes and thrombocytes or cases where more transfusions are expected in the future. The use of filtrated or washed erythrocytes is necessary in these cases to avoid discomfort to the patient and wastage of blood of which transfusion could not be completed. In this respect the hospital staff must define a transfusion reaction, and criteria for the use of the blood components should be developed. As a good example Goldfinger and Lowe (14) in a recent study on the incidence of transfusion reactions proved the advantage of washed erythrocytes and gave some recommendation for their use.

On the other hand the medical staff must realize that there are some disadvantages in using blood components. Washing of erythrocytes before administration will increase costs; and, because a closed system is opened, the erythrocytes must be used within a certain time.

If filtrated or washed erythrocytes are used in the proper way, fewer febrile transfusion reactions will be seen than in situations wherein this procedure is not followed. The percentage of febrile reactions therefore can be used as a parameter of good transfusion practice, and the medical staff can develop an outcome criterium for this complication.

The quality assurance of the preparation of blood components is beyond the scope of evaluation of the bloodtransfusion practice in hospitals: it is the responsibility of the blood bank and laboratory.

THE SUPPLY MANAGEMENT AND OUTDATING OF BLOOD

When there exists a surplus of units of blood in an assigned or cross-matched status, it will take much time between donation and administration of blood and thus the age of the erythrocytes will increase. As a disadvantage especially in patients with chronic anaemia these red cells having a shorter in vivo survival may lead to more frequent transfusions. Moreover, when more cross-matches than necessary are done, costs as well as the chance of mistakes will increase. For the use of blood in the operating room, the establishing of a maximum surgical blood order schedule, including type-and-screen strategy, can be of great help in achieving good supply management (15). Therefore the medical staff must calculate how many units blood are used in common surgical procedures in their hospital. With this number a list of really necessary units of blood that must be in the reserve status, can be determined. A low ratio of cross-matched versus transfused blood (CT-ratio) will indicate that few units blood are in the assigned status. The medical staff must develop criteria for an optimal CT-ratio, for an acceptable age of administrated erythrocytes and for an acceptable percentage of outdated erythrocytes.

THE REGISTRATION AND TREATMENT OF COMPLICATIONS

After any given bloodtransfusion, a complication can occur. Therefore, guidelines must be present about how to deal with a transfusion reaction. Distinction must be made between treatment of these complications and measures for investigation of the cause of the complication after the event. Complications must be registered so as to facilitate the identification of causes, the prevention of similar reactions, to measure the frequency of complications and to determine if treatment was correct. This applies also to the long-term complications such as hepatitis.

WHAT ARE WE GOING TO MEASURE

In measuring the quality of bloodtransfusion practice, most of the criteria are applied to the process of care, notably those mentioned in the section on indications and blood component therapy. The presence of guidelines for treatment of complications will meet a criterium of structure of medical care, while the treatment itself is again part of the process. Outcome criteria refer to the age of administered erythrocytes and percentage of outdated blood. As stated above, the percentage complications can be used as an outcome criterium for good medical care. The condition of the patient or his hemoglobin value after the bloodtransfusion can also be considered as an outcome criterium.

It is not necessary to measure all the mentioned items of all transfused units in all the departments of the hospital. The medical audit committee must focus attention on that part of the blood transfusion practice that may or probably will have shortcomings. As an important point to keep in mind for gathering the data to determine the use of proper indications and the use of the proper blood components, the medical staff has to investigate each transfusion individually. For such items as CT-ratio, age of administered erythrocytes, outdating of blood and percentage complications, it is possible to gather the data automatically and make analyses over an agreed interval in time.

FURTHER CONDITIONS FOR IMPROVING BLOODTRANSFUSION PRACTICE

If the practice of bloodtransfusion therapy has not met the criteria, changes in the medical care will have to be introduced. Such changes can be educational efforts of changes in the manner of requesting blood. The way of improvement depends on the sort of shortcoming and will be different for each hospital.

The medical audit committee has a great part to play in all these activities. However, the involved physicians have to develop their own criteria. If medical staff runs into problems in establishing guidelines and criteria, they can get help. In 1979 in The Netherlands a central organization for quality assurance (CBO) was established to stimulate and advise quality assurance activities in all Dutch hospitals. Within this organization, there exists a scientific council that consists of representatives of all specialties in clinical medicine. It has the main task of advising about the development and application of criteria. Recently, the CBO has organized a consensus development meeting on bloodtransfusion practice, in a joint venture with the blood banks, transfusion laboratories and clinical experts.*

* Consensus bijeenkomst: Richtlijnen voor het bloedtransfusie beleid in ziekenhuizen. CBO, Amsterdam 1982.

VALIDITY OF STRUCTURED QUALITY ASSURANCE

The literature contains only a few studies in which an improvement in bloodtransfusion practice is described. Graham-Stewart (1), Diethrich (2) and Friedman (3) published the results of a survey on blood usage, but they gave no re-assessment after the introduction of a change. Okuno and Nelson (11) described a steady decline of single-unit transfusion over 11 years but it coincided with an upsurge of public interest and not with the provision of appropriate information to the medical staff. Powell and Johnston (12) showed that after education efforts in hospital meetings the percentage of non-indicated single unit transfusions decreased from 80% to 52%. Mc Coy (6) reported the results of a survey over 7 years: after the adoption of "indications for bloodtransfusion" by the medical staff the units transfused per patient declined from 0.237 to 0.110 in his hospital. In our hospital we have done two studies on the practice of blood usage. In 1977 we described (16) an increase in use of packed cells from 25% to 70% after introduction of an educational effort and, more importantly, after changing the form by which blood and blood component have to be requested; whole blood as such was not mentioned anymore on this form. Recently (4) we described a study on the indications of bloodtransfusion. Criteria for the indications for transfusion of patients with chronic anaemia, post-operative anaemia and acute blood loss were developed by an internist, a surgeon and an anesthesist. During two months, every transfusion was evaluated separately by the same physicians who had established the criteria. The indication as well as the amount of units of blood given were judged. After the survey an educational effort was made. In the second survey one year later, there was found a decrease from 23% to 9% in unjustified transfusions.

CONCLUSIONS

Bloodtransfusion practice is a suitable topic for structured quality assurance. The medical staff and especially the involved physicians must develop advice and guidelines regarding the four mentioned items. If possible, explicit criteria based on the available literature must be established. However, under some circumstances such as the establishment of indications for the transfusion, implicit judgment will be necessary. Other aspects of blood transfusion practice such as CT-ratio and percentage of complications can be monitored.

The practice of bloodtransfusion therapy must be measured against the explicit and implicit criteria and if shortcomings are found, a change in medical care delivery must be introduced. The medical staff needs a quality assurance committee that can ascertain what aspects of the bloodtransfusion practice must be measured and can coordinate all activities towards this purpose.

In The Netherlands, the Scientific Council of the CBO can help such a quality assurance committee in establishing these criteria.

ACKNOWLEDGMENT

I thank J. Hudson MD, staff-member of the CBO, for his critical remarks and advice in the preparation of this manuscript.

REFERENCES

1. Grahm-Stewart, C.W. A clinical survey of bloodtransfusion. Lancet 1960;ii:421–4.
2. Diethrich, E.G. Evaluation of bloodtransfusion therapy. Transfusion of nonoperated anemic patients. Transfusion 1978; 18:193–8.
4. Baarveld, F., Lopes Cardozo, M., Russchen C.J., Thomas, Th.A., Casparie, A.F. Intercollegiale toetsing in een ziekenhuis: toepassing van vaste en persoonlijke criteria in een onderzoek naar de indicaties van bloodtransfusies. Ned. Tijdsch. Geneesk. 1982;126:1717–20.
5. Wintrobe, M.M. Clinical hematology. 8th ed. Philadelphia: Lea and Febiger 1981;491–519.
6. Mc Coy, K.I. The providence hospital blood conservation program. Transfusion 1962;2:3–5.
7. Crosby, W.H. Misuse of bloodtransfusion. Blood 1958;13:1198–1200.
8. Abdulla, W., Frey, R., Witzke. Empfehlungen zur Transfusion-therapy. Münch. med. Wschr. 1979;121:1051–4.
9. Morton, J.H. An evaluation of bloodtransfusion practices on a surgical service. N. Engl. J. Med. 1960;263:1285–7.
10. Gibbs, C.E., Misenhimer, H.R. The use of bloodtransfusions in obstetrics. Am. J. Obstet. Gynecol. 1965;93:26–31.
11. Okuno, T., Nelson, A. Recent trends of blood usage in a suburgan general hospital. Ill. med. J. 1975;147:63–6.
12. Powell, N.A., Johnston, D.G. Criteria for bloodtransfusions. Calif medicine 1962;87:12–5.
13. Bear, R.W. Recommendations concerning the indications for the use of blood and blood products. Pathology 1978;10:177–9.
14. Goldfinger, D., Lowe, C. Prevention of adverse reactions to bloodtransfusion by the administration of saline-washed red blood cells. Transfusion 1981;21:277–80.
15. Friedman, B.A., Oberman, H.A., Chadwick, A.R., Kingdon, A.R. The maximum surgical blood order schedule and surgical blood use in the United States. Transfusion 1976;16:380–7.
16. Casparie, A.F., Reerink, E. Intercollegiale toetsing in een ziekenhuis: het selectieve gebruik van "packed cells" voor transfusie als onderwerp van prospectieve kwaliteitsbewaking. Ned. Tijdsch. Geneesk. 1977;120:55–9.

DISCUSSION

Moderators: H.F. Taswell, J.W. Dorpema

Chairman: Thank you Dr. Casparie for the very interesting presentation on this subject, which is extremely important and frequently felt to be out of the hands of the blood banker, but I do believe we should have that attitude. We have to take the approach that you have described.

C.F. Högman, Uppsala, Sweden:

I have one first comment to Dr. Leikola about the ISBT guides. I was not aware of the fact that they sold out completely, because they have been reprinted. I think there is a need for these guides, for instance, the quality assurance guide. Requests should be submitted to the ISBT for further reprinting.

Another more general remark is about the definitions. One problem we have in the bloodtransfusion services is that several of the products are so very poorly defined, as far as quality goes. For instance, I cannot think of anything less defined than whole blood, particularly if you disregard its age. The easiest way to get around this problem is to completely abolish whole blood. It would clear things up considerably in the minds of the clinicians if whole blood were no longer available. This is actually what has been done in my own hospital, as it has been done in several other hospitals also. The main advantage is that you can actually stress quality. For instance, one can emphasize the possibility of decreasing the frequency of febrile reactions by about 80% when removing the buffy coat cells, and also all the plasma from the red cells to make it a red cell suspension instead. This makes it possible to reduce the use of plasma in elective surgery by about 75 to 80%, which makes plasma available for fractionation.

The point of this remark is that we can achieve very much by stressing the quality of the products and defining them. Now, one difficulty is that we define several products by the way we treat them, for instance washed red cells, buffy coat poor red cells and so forth. It would be far better to define the quality of the product instead of describing how it was treated. We could define for instance like micro-aggregate-poor red cells, or micro-aggregate and plasma-poor red cells, which would probably tell

carrying capacity of the lost or hemolysed red cells has to be replaced. In chronic anaemias due to the well known compensatory mechanisms a dynamic equilibrium is attained at much lower levels of hemoglobin.

My other comment is: you mentioned some limits in pre-operative anaemia. I would like to add something to this, that the majority of wasted blood is wasted in operating-theaters. We have to stress to surgeons the fact that they do not really need a certain fixed level of hemoglobin, because the healing of the wound or the recovery of the patient will not exclusively depend on this. However, we have to stress also that giving whole blood 48 hours before the operation, just to correct the hemoglobin level, is a dangerous practice. Leucocytes will be destroyed in the lungs and so respiratory distress syndrome may eventually occur. Most of those patients who are anaemic before an elective operation are in fact iron-deficient. It would be much safer for the patient and much better for the bloodtransfusion service, if they would send these patients back, prepare them through effective iron medication and operate in elective surgery after two or three months.

In brief, there are two possibilities for coping with the misuse of whole blood. The first one is the autocratic method mentioned. I have always been against autocratic methods, as these alone will not help. One can get a very rapid result but I agree with Dr. van der Does that the results will not be firm, because those physicians and surgeons who are obsessed by the myth of whole blood will put together blood in a more expensive form.

So, I think priority should be given to post-graduate teaching and constant and continuous consultation between hospitals and Blood Banks, as the only method with which we can yield long-term success against the misuse of blood.

J. Leikola, Geneva, Switzerland:

I would like to add a couple of comments to Dr. Högman's remarks. One concerns the names of the products, when you are referring to washed red cells and filtrated red cells. This is quite appropriate. I think it is the responsibility of the clinician to know what is in the product. When you give a definition to a product, it is up to the clinician to know the composition of the product. However, it is up to the Blood Bank to teach the clinicians, as it is up to the pharmacologists to teach the clinicians how to administer drugs and medicines.

Secondly you mentioned that whole blood is very poorly defined. This is quite true, but the patient is also very poorly defined, as is the loss of blood. What is meant by this? We are dealing with fairly abstract concepts. In my mind, I think that whole blood will keep its definite place in transfusion therapy. Instead of building up a system in which whole blood has no place, in order to procure more plasma, the voluntary plasmapheresis should be increased, where red cells are given back to the donor.

Chairman: I will take the chairman's prerogative for a comment and stress a few comments that were made. One is that we all know that changes have to be made. We strive for them. But I would have to agree that they should not be achieved by dictatorial methods. Even if it takes longer, they have to come about by evolution and by education by techniques, such as modifying transfusion request forms, which bring about the changes in subtle ways.

The second point is that while we frequently look down on the practice of some clinician or surgeon and say: "They are using whole blood in such and such situation, with no valid reason". Let us not fall into the same trap of arrogance that they might be in. Remember what Dr. Casparie pointed out: there is really nothing in the literature to give us firm information about when we should transfuse or what should be transfused. So we as blood bankers are standing on very shaky ground ourselves. I do not think we should be too absolute and certain about our own absolute correctness.

As a last point I would like to ask a question to Dr. Casparie and the audience. How do you think we can approach this problem? You mention that there is variation in the literature as to what is an appropriate hemoglobin, and, if so, how can we go about putting criteria on indications for transfusions on some firm basis, a firmer basis than the surgeon and the blood banker now have?

A.F. Casparie:

I think this a very important question, but a difficult one to answer. What to do should be with regard to prospects: whether you transfuse some patients and others not, what the results are when you transfuse patients after and/or during operation. More is known about the hematocrit and hemodilution, where it is not necessary to have a normal hematocrit during operation. But it is going to be very difficult clinical research to define when a transfusion is needed.

Ch.A. Schiffer, Baltimore, USA:

I would not dare to insert myself into the whole-blood/packed-cells controversy. However, it seems to me that data ought to be available because there are an enormous number of institutions, particularly in the United States, that essentially do nothing but transfuse packed cells. That includes our hospital which has a major cancer centre, and probably one of the larger trauma centres in the country, if not the world. They utilize almost exclusively packed cells plus supplementation of albumin when necessary. That may not answer the question, but at least it gives you the data to answer the question in terms of what the relative costs of this approach are. There is no doubt that one can get away with packed cells in the overwhelming majority of cases. The question is how much whole blood do you have to have around?

I would like to comment, however, on the necessity for eliminating the buffy coat from packed cells or bloodtransfusion. It is obvious that the patient does not need the buffy coat. That is not the issue. But in our hospital, the various ways of removing the buffy coat do double or treble the cost of the unit. They also make it that the unit outdates within 24 hours. For surgical considerations, a lot of the blood that is ordered does not get used, and, conceivably, some of the blood that you modify for those patients would have to be outdated as well.

I guess the figures of how many people have trouble with transfusion reactions are available. It is clearly the small minority of patients. Exceptions are patients who are on repeated transfusion programs, such as would exist in a cancer centre. Our patients in the cancer centre do not all develop transfusion reactions. The minority of those patients do. We find it a reasonable cost-effective policy to utilize packed cells for those patients and then switch to the washed product, which is what our Blood Bank provides at the time the transfusion reactions develop. We have thought a great deal about this and find that this represents the most cost-effective and logical approach for us.

Chairman: I would like to give everyone at least one chance to speak before we return to anyone who has a second or third comment.

R.J. Crawford, Glasgow, Scotland:

In answer to Dr. Hollán, I feel it is useful to teach clinicians that the place of blood for transfusion to cover elective surgery is on a shelf in the refrigerator, and not in the patient. This does stop quite a lot of transfusion reactions, and each donation helps a lot more patients. Also, it turns you around and it becomes an active, conscious decision to say "My goodness, here is a patient who actually could benefit from a transfusion", as opposed to "The blood loss looks like a liter, let's give him a transfusion".

Chairman: Said like a true Scotsman!

R.J. Crawford:

Another point is the reconstituted not quite whole blood. We keep stocks of red cell concentrate, of fresh frozen plasma and platelets. We believe that CPD red cell concentrate stores quite happily at 4°C for a while. Plasma has to be frozen. Good platelets are kept at 20°C in a special agitator. Keep them all in their perfect condition; do not reconstitute them. Once you have got each component stored as it should be, preferably transfuse separately rather than have bags of confusing material, which is a buffy-coat-poor, platelet-poor not exactly whole blood, with the plasma deteriorating. So, I believe in keeping separate stocks of each component, recombining by prescription at the bedside in the patient.

J.A. Loos, Amsterdam, The Netherlands:

Dr. Taswell, is it not necessary to define your product as a measure of quality control also? I want to support Dr. Högman in his statement. All the ignorance regarding the effects of different products comes from the fact that the clinicians who use the different products do not exactly know what they are using, because the labels do not specify the constituents. I think one of the most important aspects of quality control is that it should lead to a definition of the product.

Chairman: I would accept that as a very valid suggestion and criticism. Dr. Högman's suggestion of the need to define products is a very excellent one. I would agree.

C.F. Högman:

I intentionally made my comment provocative in order to raise a discussion. Just to make things fully clear: I am also for evolution and not for revolution. I would like to stress that what we really need is a two-way communication between the clinicians and the Blood Bank, to provide them with data about the nature and properties of our products. It is our duty to collect this data, which relates very much to the subject of this conference, namely that we should try to define the quality of our different products. This would enable us to arrive at a statement that whole blood is extremely poorly defined.

One further comment. When one needs whole blood, one usually needs a lot, even when it puts the Blood Bank in a very awkward situation, particularly when it has to be very fresh. This is why, from a logistical point of view it might be much better to go in for a component therapy program. In this case, you could say: "Instead of whole blood, you could use these and these products". This would be a simple solution for those who are using these products.

Chairman: I would like to close with one comment. Although we look with suspicion at the practices of our clinical colleagues, we have to remember that they are at the bedside of the patient, and with the primary responsibility for the care and for the life of that patient. While sometimes their experience or their practice may be anecdotal we also have to give them the benefit of the doubt. Although their experience may be anecdotal, it may be correct. We have to recognize that much of our experience is perhaps anecdotal, and without a solid scientific basis. So, let us be fair. Let us not be too absolute. Let us try to collect the information needed for a reasonable scientific decision, and in the meantime try to do the best we can without falling into the same kind of mistakes that we see and are so critical of.

II. Systems and procedures

PRINCIPLES AND PRACTICES OF QUALITY CONTROL

F. Bonanni

INTRODUCTION

Industry in general is a positive element of society, that contributes to the improvement of the human condition in a variety of ways, by supplying needed goods and services, by distributing wealth to investors and by creating environments where people can realize themselves fully. Industry has a value to society that goes beyond the generation of profit. Profit is only a tangible measure of how society appreciates the value contributed by a specific company.

In no other field are these features as obvious as in the pharmaceutical industry. The value of the pharmaceutical industry to society is the supply of safe and effective products for use by the medical community in providing health care. Keywords here are "safe" and "effective". While nobody would knowingly distribute products that might hurt a patient, rather than cure him or her, today's reality of mass production is that a manufacturing process may yield, statistically, a number of defective units. The likelihood of a process to yield defective products can be controlled, i.e. monitored and kept within acceptable limits, through a series of measures collectively known as the quality control program.

The notion of quality is central to the pharmaceutical industry, which can only maximize its value to society by improving the quality of its products and services, and by developing new valuable products and services.

Hence the fundamental communality of interests and goals between professionals in the health care industry and professionals in the medical community.

For quality to be present at the point of use of a pharmaceutical product, it has to be present in each phase of a product life cycle. Such a cycle includes design, research and development, manufacturing and distribution. Quality as fitness for use is the end result of how well a product is designed in the first place, how well developed it is, how well it is manufactured and ultimately made available to the user (Figure 1).

To keep this presentation within reasonable limits, I will focus on some key aspects of quality control, which is that portion of the quality assurance program dealing with quality of conformance of the manufacturing process to agreed-upon specifications and standards.

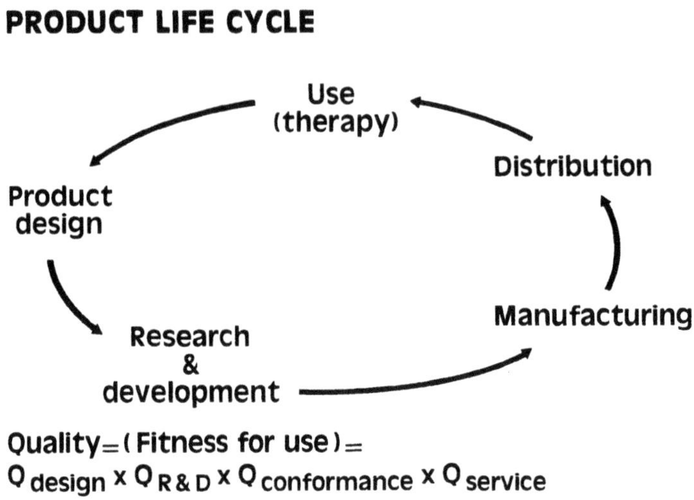

Figure 1. Product life cycle.

DISCUSSION

QUALITY CONTROL ASPECTS IN THE MANUFACTURE OF PLASTIC BAGS FOR THE COLLECTION, PRESERVATION AND ADMINISTRATION OF BLOOD AND BLOOD COMPONENTS

An overal view of the manufacturing process of a brand of blood bags of wide-spread use in Europe and elsewhere is given in Figures 2 and 3. This manufacturer has chosen to have a vertically integrated process, i.e. a process that includes all phases of manufacturing, including plastic processing and plastification of PVC, up to and excluding polymerization of vinyl chloride itself.

Vertical integration lends itself ideally to the application of a total quality control program that covers all manufacturing steps. In such an approach, quality can effectively be built into the product at each step, in harmony with the ultimate objective of fitness for use at the patient's bed-side.

Elements of the quality control program (QC) are listed in Figure 4. Most of these are well-known activities, and the titles are self-explanatory.

Worth noticing here, is that the QC program is a company-wide activity reflecting the organization's commitment to quality, and not simply the concern of the QC department. Purchasing departments are for instance closely involved in the vendor assurance program; research and development (R&D), manufacturing and engineering will work with QC in validating key processes, as will be discussed later; manufacturing and engineering are involved with in-process controls and with systems controls. Most departments will be involved in personnel training, while laboratory controls are indeed a typical QC activity.

In all this the information services or EDP department assists in providing mechanized ways to store data, to analyze it statistically and to retrieve it according to various criteria, when necessary. In the more advanced companies today, applications of computer technology extend into interactive process controls and into robotics with potential quantum jumps in overall quality assurance and in reliability.

Going back to the manufacturing process flow for blood bags, the next figures illustrate certain details of the production process and outline key elements of the QC program as it applies to them.

FENWAL PROCESS FLOW (1)

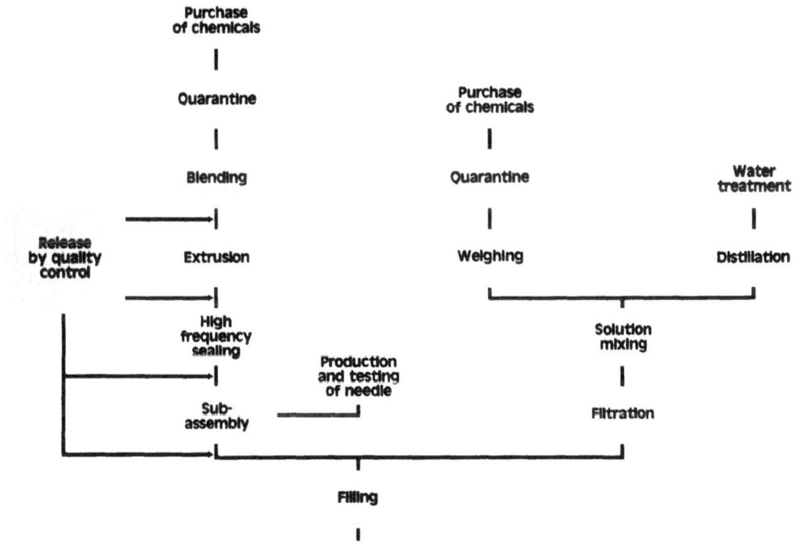

Figure 2

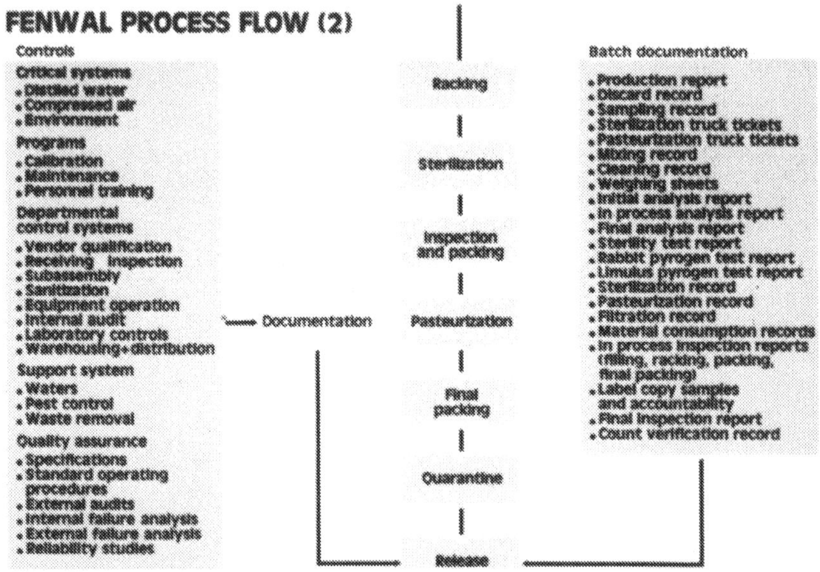

Figure 3

Figures 5, 6 and 7 show the manufacturing process flows for componentry, chemical preparation and further processing, respectively.

Key to the achievement of final quality at the patient's bed-side, is indeed the ability to perform each step in the process with a consistently high degree of conformance to established specifications. Obviously, this same principle will also apply to the manipulations and processes that take place in the medical environment, both at the blood bank and in the hospital ward.

But equally key to the achievement of ultimate product quality is a process of relatively recent introduction, to which I have referred constantly in the past few figures. This is the notion of validation, which in my opinion is central to the concept of good manufacturing practice, and which is of special importance in conjunction with the advent of computerization, automation and robotics.

In fact, validation is essential if these modern technologies are to represent a progress in quality assurance and not just an industrial engineer's dream of reduced labor costs.

ELEMENTS OF THE QUALITY CONTOL PROGRAM OF A VERTICALLY INTEGRATED MANUFACTURER OF BLOOD COLLECTION UNITS

• Vendor assurance program	vendor validation, receiving inspection trend evaluation
• Validation of key processes	
• In-process controls	
• Systems contol	water air environment facilities
• Personnel training	
• Laboratory controls	chemistry mechanical - physical microbiology pyrogens
• Calibrations, metrology	
• Audits	
• Documentation	specifications records

Figure 4

My ancestors craftsmen in renaissance Florence did not have quality control departments, and most people today will agree with me that they did not need them (a notorious exception in the family is Bonanno Pisano, architect of the Pisa tower, who linked

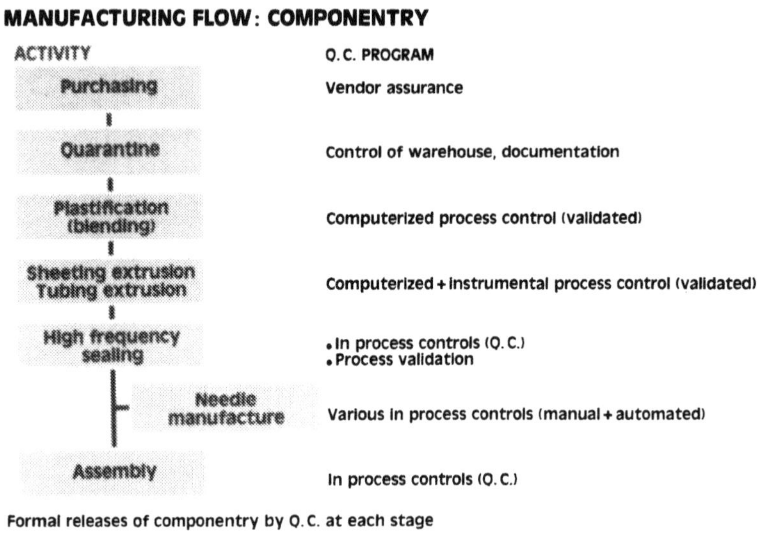

Figure 5

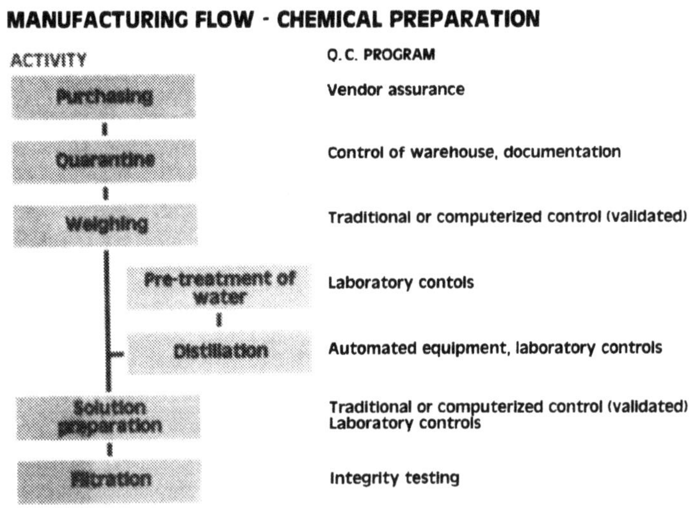

Figure 6

MANUFACTURING FLOW: PROCESSING

ACTIVITY	Q.C. PROGRAM
Filling	Traditional or computerized controls (validated) - Laboratory controls
Sterilization	Validation, Automated + manual controls Laboratory controls
Inspection & packing	100% testing + statistical Q.C.
Pasteurization	Validation, Automated + manual controls Laboratory controls
Packing	In process controls (Q.C.)
Quarantine	Documentation proofing and reconciliation Control of warehouse
Release to Distribution	Traceability

Figure 7

architecture with a genius for advertising). The industrial revolution and subsequent social events brought about a deepening rift, an alienation between man and the result of his work. This was to be exasperated by the early attempts at automation, which further dissociated the worker from his creation. In this context, the introduction of quality control systems and technologies has been a necessary and successful endeavor, balancing off the unfortunate dissociation between worker and work.

Recent developments in management techniques, are trying to reunite man and the result of his work and in particular to give back to each worker, with the dignity that is his, the notion that his input as an individual is irreplaceable, especially when it comes to quality and to creativity. Typical examples of this evolution are programs such as quality circles and quality of worklife which stress the impact of participative management on quality.

At the advanced point where we are today in the pursuit of excellence in quality, it would be a step backward to assume that more quality will come for free with further progresses of electronics, automation and robotics. Contrary to most men, a robot can be wrong 100% of the time unless its operation has been thoroughly validated.

To validate a manufacturing process means to demonstrate experimentally that such a process yields consistently a product corresponding to specifications, under a variety of operating conditions.

When validating a process, one typically identifies first the critical parameters of such a process, which can influence specified product characteristics. One then studies the acceptable ranges of values for such parameters, which still yield acceptable products. These ranges will be known as operating windows.

In the course of a validation, a process may be challenged with specific limit conditions, to further verify the correctness of the statistical tools employed and reproduce extreme "real life" situations.

As an example of a validation process in the manufacture of blood bags, I would like to illustrate the validation of sterilization as it is applied at the manufacturer which we have used as a reference so far.

A world-wide accepted standard for the sterility of terminally sterilized pharmaceutical products is the presence of not-more-than one contaminated unit in one million of units produced. A definition such as this is necessary since sterility, as absence of viable microorganisms, is a probability function and not an absolute concept. The degree of sterility achieved by a sterilization cycle in a population of objects, such as a collection of blood bags, depends on the heat exposure, on the number of microorganisms present or bioburden, and on the heat resistance of those microorganisms. The critical parameters of the sterilization process are listed in Figure 8.

CRITICAL PARAMETERS
OF THE STERILIZATION PROCESS

Bioburden	**quantity, heat resistance characteristics**
Temperature	**distribution in the vessel penetration inside the product**
Pressure	
Time	

Figure 8

As we know from basic microbiology, the surviving proportion of a pure microbial population exposed to a lethal temperature is an exponential function of the time of exposure to such a temperature. Figure 9 illustrates this relationship.

These curves are determined experimentally by exposing a pure culture to a constant lethal temperature for varying amounts of time, and determining the number of survivor organisms.

For a given microbial strain, the inactivation or death rate depends on the temperature: the higher the temperature, the faster the rate. The mathematical expression of this relationship is again exponential, and fits a first order reaction kinetic model. The two parameters appearing in these formulas, the decimal reduction rate or D and Z, are typical of each microbial strain.

Real life situations differ from the picture presented above in two ways. First, bioburden is rarely, if ever, composed of a pure microbial population but is rather a mixture of species or strains. The logarithmic death rate function applies to each population independently, the most resistent one determining the overall probability of survival.

Second, the physics of heat transfer within a sterilization vessel will determine a continuous succession of temperatures within the product during the cycle. An example of this is shown in Figure 10.

INFLUENCE OF TEMPERATURE ON DEATH RATES

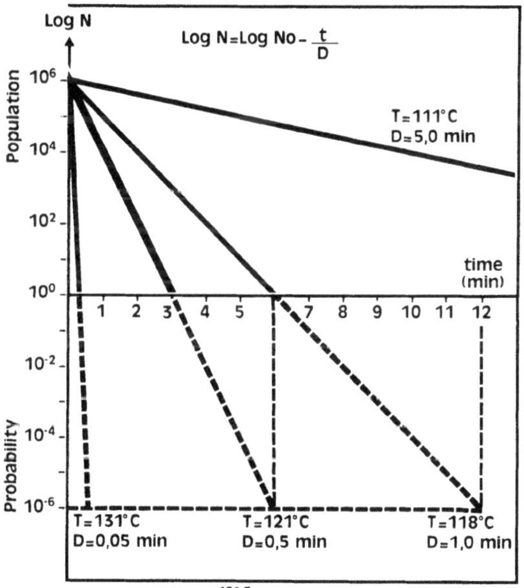

$$D = D(T) = D(121) . 10^{\frac{121-T}{Z}}$$

Z=increase in temperature necessary to reduce D by 90%

Figure 9

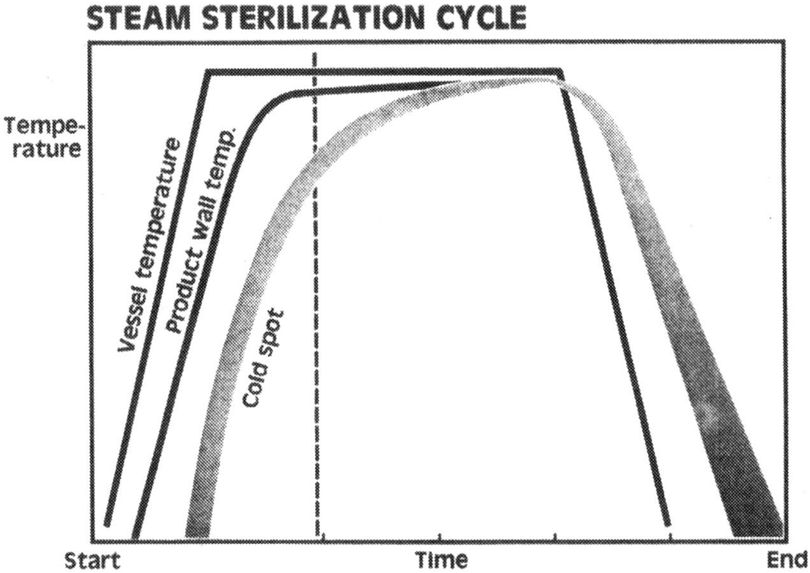

Figure 10

BASIC MATHEMATICS OF STERILIZATION

At constant temperature (T) above 100°C, for a pure microbial population:

$$\text{Log } N = \text{Log } N_o - \frac{t}{D}$$

where $D(T) = D(T_o) \cdot 10^{\frac{T_o - T}{z}}$

By taking as reference conditions $T_o = 121.1°C$ and $z = 10°C$, Fo is defined as:

$$F_o = \sum_{cycle} 10^{\frac{T-121.1}{10}} . \Delta t \quad \text{or:} \quad \int_{T=100°}^{T=100°} 10^{\frac{T-121.1}{10}} dt$$

For a sterilization cycle, we have:

$$\text{Log } N = \text{Log } N_o - \frac{F_o}{D(121.1)}$$

or =

$$(\text{Assurance of sterility}) = (\text{Bioburden}) - \frac{(\text{Lethality})}{(\text{Resistance})}$$

Figure 11

While the vessel wall has a temperature profile close to a square-wave, reaching rapidly the exposure temperature, the coldest spot of the load, inside the product, experiences a gradual increase in temperature. Still, any fraction of time spent at temperature above 100°C has a lethal effect on the bioburden. The overall lethal effect of the cycle is the integration of all lethal contributions at temperatures above 100°C.

Mathematically, the lethality of a sterilization cycle is expressed in terms of Fo, or equivalent minutes at 121.1°C. The definition of Fo is summarized in Figure 11. Maintaining the product at 121.1°C for Fo minutes would be as lethal as the actual sterilization cycle concerned. Formally, Fo is expressed in minutes and replaces the time in the logarithmic death rate expression, when the temperature is variable. Fo can be measured experimentally for each cylce by using temperature probes inside the product and recording the temperature profile throughout the cycle.

To validate a sterilization cycle means to demonstrate experimentally that its lethality is consistently capable of yielding an acceptable assurance of sterility when applied to actual bioburdens or to selected biological indicator organisms.

A method used by the reference manufacturer to validate the sterilization of blood bags in a European plant will be presented here in general terms. A detailed description is being published elsewhere.

The first step of this study consisted in measuring the bioburden levels experienced in blood bags before sterilization. Then, loads of blood bags were exposed to sterilization cycles of different duration.

The number of survivor organisms were counted at the end of each fractional exposure. The same process was repeated for blood bags inoculated with known quantities of a calibrated biological indicator organism (Bacillus subtilis 5230). Inocula of 10^6 spores of B I were placed in the anticoagulant, in the transfer

SUMMARY OF MICROBIOLOGICAL RESULTS FOR FRACTIONAL EXPOSURE STUDIES FOR SINGLE PACK BLOOD BAGS

Test unit	Mean bioburden and B.I. control counts (CFU)	Mean survivors/unit for fractional exposures of % of cycle					
		0.25%	12.5%	25.0%	37.5%	50.0%	100%
Solution bioburden	3.1	0	0	0	0	0	0
Solution biological indicator	$3.8 \cdot 10^6$	$1.8 \cdot 10^6$	$4.8 \cdot 10^5$	$2.4 \cdot 10^4$	$3.6 \cdot 10^1$	$1.4 \cdot 10^0$	0
Tab biological indicator	$2.5 \cdot 10^6$	$1.9 \cdot 10^6$	$1.61 \cdot 10^5$	$1.7 \cdot 10^3$	$9.5 \cdot 10^1$	$0.5 \cdot 10^0$	0
Transfer tube biological indicator	$2.2 \cdot 10^6$	$2.9 \cdot 10^5$	$1.6 \cdot 10^4$	$2.3 \cdot 10^2$	$3.2 \cdot 10^0$	$0.1 \cdot 10^0$	0

Figure 12

tube and in the access port known as a "tab". The latter two positions were tested to verify that sterility was achieved even in conditions of varying moisture content (i.e. water activity): experience indicates that microorganisms exhibit significant changes in heat resistance at different water activities.

Biological indicator organisms are used when, as in this case, the natural bioburden is too low in numbers to allow measurements of survivors after fractional cycle exposures. Figure 12 summarizes the results of this study.

The actual bioburden is reported in this study as having a maximum heat resistance measured historically of less than 0.2 minutes at 121.1°C (D 121.1).

If for the sake of argument, one imagines that the bioburden is composed rather than a heat-sensitive organisms, as in actuality, of heat resistance spores of characteristics similar to the biological indicator (i.e. D(121.1°) = 0.5 min, Z = 6.6°C), the resulting death rate during a sterilization cycle is shown in Figure 13.

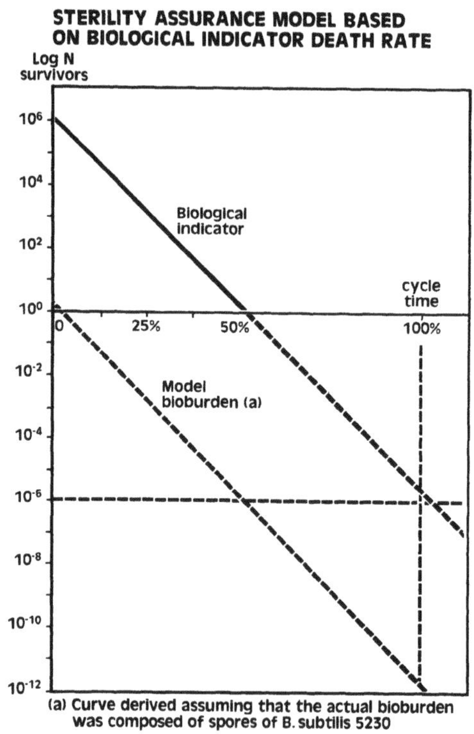

Figure 13

This study demonstrates that with naturally occurring bioburdens, the assurance of sterility achieved at the end of this sterilization cycle is many orders of magnitude beyond the accepted goal of 10^{-6}. The study also proves that portions of the bag with more difficult access of steam are sterilized as effectively or more effectively than the anticoagulant solution.

Conversely, one could use this type of validation study to tailor sterilization conditions to the actual bioburden experienced, with the goal of providing a sterility assurance greater than 10^{-6}. This may be warranted in the presence of heat labile substances, where one needs to limit the degradation caused by heat exposure. Figure 14 illustrates such an approach.

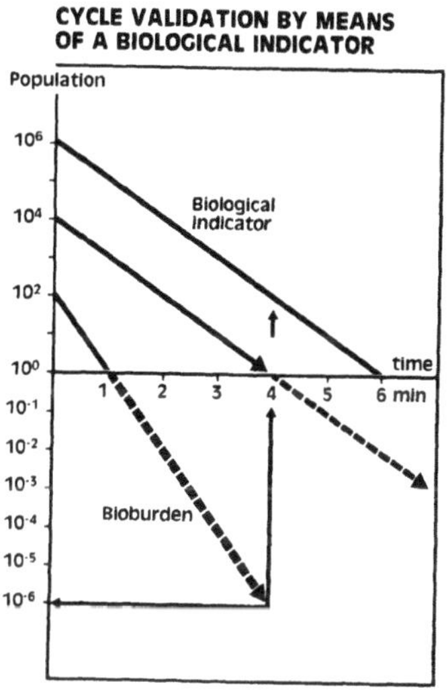

Figure 14

As a measure of internal validity for this study, the actual spore logarithm reduction rates obtained in the sterilizer for the biological indicator were compared against those calculated from the physical F values measured, and a good agreement was found.

In a validation program, the sterilization quality engineer also demonstrates that the design lethality, or Fo, is always delivered to the product. This is done through heat penetration studies, that measure the temperature profiles within the product itself, in several positions within the load, in various geometries and loading patterns.

The quality engineer will also demonstrate that the process is reproducible when all parameters operate within the specified windows. A safety factor is then added by using as a reference the slowest-heating zone in the product.

Indeed the state-of-the-art for sterility assurance within the pharmaceutical industry has come a long way since the days when the sterility test was the only method to measure it. With the high level of concern for good manufacturing practice at our reference manufacturer, most batches would pass the sterility test already before sterilization.*

I hope this single example of validation will suffice to render adequately the depth of commitment to quality of the pharmaceutical industry.

I will conclude by commenting on one element of the overall quality program that lays at the interface between the manufacturer of blood bags and the blood bank and which is, in my opinion, of great importance in assuring quality at the patient's bed-side.

I am referring here to the feed-back of performance information from the blood bank to the manufacturer. Blood bags have the unique characteristic among pharmaceutical products of being a raw material, a component in the highly complex process of collecting, fractionating, preserving, and administering a precious, living human tissue, blood.

And this process is highly diversified according to the practices in use at a specific blood bank, to its logistics requirements, its size, the wealth of its resources etc. Even within a single blood bank the process variables are numerous ranging from the inherent individual donor characteristics, to the use of mobile collection units, to the presence of different equipment, to personnel turnover, to seasonal fluctuations.

I have been personally involved recently in a collaborative study with a major European blood bank aimed at defining a comprehensive quality assurance program which includes the validation of key processes. I can report that such a task is highly complex and will require extensive, skilled work to reach its completion.

In this context, it is extremely important for the blood bank to study the performance characteristics of blood bags in detail under its unique operating conditions, and to report them methodically to the manufacturer. Conversely, it is highly desirable if not essential in this field that the manufacturer operates an active service organization to gather such reports from the blood banks and to act on them to improve performance characteristics, when necessary.

In the age of computers and robotics this notion of human communication and interface may appear trivial. In my opinion it is the single area likely to yield the most results in terms of quality improvement and general product innovation, at this point in time, if properly addressed.

* Still, the sterility test is the only analytical method available to the Authorities to verify the sterility of a product.

BLOOD BANK STANDARDS AND PROCEDURE MANUALS

P.J. Schmidt

It has been the goal of the scientist who describes new things to tell us what were the methods used in observation of the results. As such new things become routine, they should also become regularly reproducible, provided that the original techniques are followed. That requires that the original description of the methods were clear and correct.

An example is the practical exercise that is provided to every class of students studying for their degree in Medicine in Tampa. You would recognize the directions as those for Landsteiner's simple cross grouping experiment on the blood of his laboratory colleagues. After their exercise is over, the students are told to think clearly and simply, and perhaps they too will win a Nobel Prize. The 1900 procedures are brief, clear and simple. The results of following those procedures eighty years later are predictable.

But the rest of us are now describing more complex things than Landsteiner's experiment. How are we to explain our systems to those who must carry them out? Since such systems involve people, they are vastly more difficult to program than computers or robots. We call our explanations Procedure Manuals, Standard Operating Procedures or Standards.

Procedure manuals can be mostly pictorial. It is to the Chinese that we attribute the saying that "one picture is worth more than ten thousand words". Certainly pictures have the great advantage of being apparent in any language. Since English is such a difficult language with such strange rules, we know that many written procedures "lose in translation". One of the regular comic episodes in America is the depiction of the man who buys the unassembled toy for his child at Christmas. He attempts to fit the toy parts together at the last moment, working from enclosed directions printed in Japan. Those directions have been translated from the Japanese idiom into English by someone who does not converse in English. Americans have enough difficulty understanding the precise English that is written in England let alone Japanese English.

If I am to talk about both Procedure Manuals and Standards, I must define them both since they are different things. By Standards, I do not mean the original specimen that sets the measure

The Operation of a
Hospital Transfusion Service

PART I—The Preservation and Transfusion of Whole Human Blood

PART II—The Processing and Use of Citrated Human Blood Plasma

OCD Publication 2220 • March 1944

Medical Division
OFFICE OF CIVILIAN DEFENSE
Washington 25, D. C.

Figure 1. The earliest American Manual of Standard Operating Procedures, 1944.

OXFORD MEDICAL PUBLICATIONS

BLOOD
TRANSFUSION

BY

VICTOR HORSLEY RIDDELL
M.A., M.D. CAMB., F.R.C.S. ENG.
Assistant Surgeon and Lecturer in Operative Surgery, St. George's Hospital, London
Assistant Surgeon, Royal Waterloo Hospital, London
Consultant British Red Cross Transfusion Service

OXFORD UNIVERSITY PRESS
LONDON : HUMPHREY MILFORD
1939

Figure 2.

OXFORD MEDICAL PUBLICATIONS

INDIVIDUALITY OF THE BLOOD

IN BIOLOGY AND IN CLINICAL AND FORENSIC MEDICINE

BY

PROFESSOR LEONE LATTES

DIRECTOR OF THE INSTITUTE OF FORENSIC MEDICINE IN THE UNIVERSITY OF MODENA

TRANSLATED BY

L. W. HOWARD BERTIE

M.A., B.M., B.Ch. (OXON.)

FROM THE FRENCH EDITION OF 1929, THOROUGHLY REVISED AND BROUGHT UP TO DATE BY THE AUTHOR

OXFORD UNIVERSITY PRESS
LONDON : HUMPHREY MILFORD
1932

Figure 3

First (Italian) edition, 1923.
German edition (revised and enlarged), 1925.
French edition (,, ,, ,,), 1929.

Figure 4. Early versions of Lattes' monograph.

of quantity, but rather the written model or statement of practice that is to be followed. The Standards, like the Ten Commandments, tell the believer what to do. On the other hand, Procedure Manuals tell the worker how to do it. Neither should discuss theory, but only practice. But also, as we shall see later, neither should they be cast into stone because the theory and the practice change for the better.

I am going to trace the historical development of two separate publications of the American Association of Blood Banks (AABB). The Technical Manual, now in its Eighth Edition, of 1981 began in 1953 as the Technical Methods and Procedures. The Standards for Blood Banks and Transfusion Services, now in its Tenth Edition, of 1981 began in 1958 as the Standards for a Blood Transfusion Service. (In 1983 the Silver Jubilee edition will be published.) Since the Technical Methods and Procedures publication antedate the Standards by five years, it would seem that things happened backwards and that we issued directions on how to do "it" before we had instructions on what to do. But in parallel fashion, it is also true that the organization of religion preceded the Ten Commandments, so that sequence is not unknown in human history.

WORLD WAR II MANUALS

The predecessors of both the Standards and Technical Manual go back to the organizational publications of World War II. Of course, all of that material is what a library accessions as Ephemera. It is transient paper material, cheaply bound, meant to be superceded and destroyed. The roots of the American materials are anchored in some now scarce wartime documents which appeared first in 1941.

In September 1941, there was printed an American Red Cross Manual, No. 784 entitled "Methods and Techniques of Blood Procurement as Prescribed by the National Research Council for Use in the Red Cross Blood Procurement Centers". It remained in effect until January 1943, when a revision called "Methods and Techniques Used in Red Cross Blood Donor Centers" was issued. The first manual was based largely on theory. The second was based on extensive practical experience (1). Of course, those manuals related to blood collection for plasma production, since World War II at its beginning was a plasma war. A manual on blood plasma was prepared in 1942 by Max Strumia for our Office of Civilian Defense (1). Our first manual on actual blood typing, cross-matching and transfusion was prepared by Elmer DeGowin for that same government agency and was published in 1944 (Figure 1). The list of references in those publications indicate that they were mostly created _de novo_ from monographs and articles in the periodical literature.

The oldest monograph reference in the DeGowin pamphlet is to Riddell's book of 1939 (Figure 2). Riddell gives a major credit to the great work by Leone Lattes which had already appeared in

BLOOD TRANSFUSION

HEMORRHAGE AND
THE ANÆMIAS

BY

BERTRAM M. BERNHEIM, A.B., M.D., F.A.C.G.
INSTRUCTOR IN CLINICAL SURGERY, THE JOHNS HOPKINS UNIVERSITY, CAPTAIN, MEDICAL OFFICERS' RESERVE CORPS, U. S. A., AUTHOR OF "SURGERY OF THE VASCULAR SYSTEM," ETC.

PHILADELPHIA AND LONDON
J. B. LIPPINCOTT COMPANY

Figure 5. The second American monograph on transfusion.

APPENDIX

CONTAINING HÆMOLYTIC AND AGGLUTINATION TESTS THAT ARE TO BE CARRIED OUT PRELIMINARY TO EVERY BLOOD TRANSFUSION EXCEPT THOSE OF THE MOST URGENT CHARACTER. THE TESTS GIVEN ARE AS FOLLOWS: (1) MOSS' METHOD OF GROUP TESTING; (2) BREM'S SIMPLIFICATION OF MOSS' GROUP METHOD; (3) SIMON'S METHOD OF TESTING OUT DONORS DIRECTLY AGAINST THE RECIPIENTS; (4) SYDENSTRICKER'S METHOD OF TESTING OUT DONORS DIRECTLY AGAINST THE RECIPIENT.

MOSS' METHOD OF GROUPING BLOODS FOR TRANSFUSION.

ACCORDING to Moss,[1] whose article on Isoagglutinins and Isohemolysins, written in 1910, still remains an undimmed landmark, all individuals can be divided into four groups as regards their blood according to the ability of their serum to agglutinate the corpuscles of other individuals, and according to the ability of their corpuscles to be agglutinated by the serum of other individuals.

[1] W. L. Moss, "Studies on Isoagglutinins and Isohemolysins." Bulletin of the Johns Hopkins Hospital, vol. xxi, No. 228, March, 1910, pp. 63–70.

233

Figure 6. Appendix to the Bernheim monograph, 1917.

English (Figure 3) and in Italian, German and French (Figure 4). Finally in this series, Lattes recognizes the 1917 monograph by Bernheim (Figure 5) of John Hopkins in Baltimore, the appendix of which contained a procedural manual (Figure 6).

1950 PROCEDURE MANUALS

Among the many workers active on the American scene during World War II was John Elliott, then of the state of North Carolina. After World War II, he moved to Miami, Florida and was involved with the combined operation of the Dade County Blood Bank and Dade Reagents. Many other workers were applying lessons learned during World War II to their own blood banks and hospitals, but the bench manuals produced on large mimeographed sheets at Dade by Elliott and his coworker, Jack Griffitts, seem to have progressed much further. Their writings became the outline of the Standard Procedures and Methods of the Florida Association of Blood Banks in 1951 (Figure 7). By 1953 and with the involvement of John B. Ross, the Technical Methods and Procedures, a first manual of the American Association of Blood Banks was produced (Figure 8).

FLORIDA ASSOCIATION OF BLOOD BANKS

Standard Procedures and Methods

INTRODUCTION

This Manual shall serve as the minimum requirements for Blood Bank operation for all member blood banks of the Florida Association of Blood Banks.

The purpose of standardization of procedures and methods is to assure the people of Florida that all member banks of the Florida Association of Blood Banks are bound by high standards in the collection and processing of blood from healthy donors in the interest of protecting not only the recipient of the blood, but also the donor of the blood and the Blood Banks.

Figure 7. The first Florida manual, 1951.

All three manuals (Dade, Florida and AABB) which date from those first few years of the 1950s share phrases and sentences in common. It is interesting to compare them and see the introduction of new ideas. For example, the earlier Florida manual has mention of neither D^u nor the antiglobulin tests – both of which are well discussed in the AABB Manual. Of course, all such improvements were due to the input of many minds from many parts of the country, who were sharing ideas with their colleagues on other continents.

That first AABB manual was a publication of both Standards plus Procedures, i.e. both what to do and how to do it. E.R. Jennings advocated that an Inspection and Accreditation program would be impossible without succinct Standards limited to just what to do. He wrote the first draft of a separate publication.

TECHNICAL

METHODS and PROCEDURES

of the

American Association of Blood Banks

Copyright 1953
by
American Association of Blood Banks
Dallas, Texas

No portion of this book may be reproduced
without the written consent of the Association.

Printed in the United States of America

Figure 8. The first AABB technical manual, 1953.

AABB STANDARDS

It is not generally known that there was a trial edition of the AABB Standards issued in 1957 (Figure 9). It was clearly marked as preliminary and was distributed to a limited number of blood bank directors with the hope they would submit suggestions (Figure 10). Some of the suggestions incorporated into the final first edition of 1958 (Figure 11) included exceptions for medical practice modifications and experimental studies.

Those early Standards show some of the problems and difficulties of change. The First Edition has this wise statement in regard to the serological test for syphilis: "the test is not required if the blood is stored for at least 96 hours prior to use". That very reasonable dictum persisted until the Fourth Edition of 1963. It has been interesting to read in Vox Sanguinis for 1981 the vehemence with which the persistence of that useless test is defended, as if we had always done it (2).

STANDARDS FOR ACCREDITATION

OF A

BLOOD TRANSFUSION SERVICE

(First Edition, 1957)

Prepared jointly by

SCIENTIFIC COMMITTEE OF THE
JOINT BLOOD COUNCIL, Inc.

and

STANDARDS COMMITTEE OF THE AMERICAN
ASSOCIATION OF BLOOD BANKS

Inquiries concerning this publication should be addressed to:

Joint Blood Council, Inc.
Chairman, Scientific Committee
1832 M Street, N.W.
Washington 6, D. C.

[redacted]

OR

American Association of Blood Banks
Chairman, Standards Committee
1211 West Washington
Phoenix, Arizona

Figure 9. The preprint of the AABB Standards, 1957.

REVISION AND IMPROVEMENT

American school children study in their English composition classes as the perfect form of essay that classic by Charles Lamb, "A Dissertation on Roast Pig". For those more interested in content rather than in form, it told a story that is applicable to the constant need for revision of Procedure Manuals, as well as Standards.

You will remember that Bo-bo was a lubberly boy who was playing with fire several thousands years ago. He burned down the family cottage and in that fire were cooked some young pigs. When he licked his seared hand, Bo-bo's incidental finding was the new and delicious flavor of roast pig. Bo-bo shared his results and procedures with the neighbors and because of that, the huts in his village burned regularly every time there was a new litter of pigs. That custom of burning dwellings grew, until the whole country was going up in flames. Finally, some sage found that it was possible to roast pig with a small, controlled fire. The new and improved procedure was drawn up and published. The villages were saved, but not the pigs. Bo-bo did the original research but the unnamed sage improved the procedure. Procedure Manuals can be changed and still result in the same product; perhaps even an improved product. Neither theory nor method are cast in stone and we must permit Bo-bo and the wise sages to improve our Standards and our Procedure Manuals.

COMPLIANCE

It would be pretentious of me to identify and list the minimum number of procedures which must be in a Manual of hospital, community blood banks or transfusion services. There are also limitations on the ideal way those Manuals, or the Standards from which they emanate, should be written.

In the United States we have two sets of Standards, we call them the double standard. One is issued by the Federal Government. Unfortunately their standards, technically called Regulations, usually drag along behind the other which are prepared by the Associations to which we belong. In one case it is the American Red Cross which concerns itself only with the donor blood. The American Association of Blood Banks has Standards for both the donor blood and the patient transfusion.

In the United States, the "responsible head" of the blood bank is charged by the government with being the one person who directs the performance of the assigned functions of employees. For blood banks and transfusion services who have voluntary accreditation from the American Association of Blood Banks, a licensed physician must direct the service in compliance with the AABB Standards.

The Standards of the AABB are not a set of directions on how to assure the quality of the product but rather a set of definitions of the goal of good practice. The dual role of the medical director

IMPORTANT NOTICE

The "Standards" in the present form is to be considered as a preliminary edition for submission to you and other workers interested in transfusion services.

This must, therefore, not be considered as a final version but should be regarded as a living, changing document subject to revision for clarification and as new and approved methods become available.

It is distributed in this version to a limited number of blood bank directors with the hope that they will submit their suggestions to the committee chairmen listed on the first page.

Figure 10. The disclaimer in the AABB Standards reprint.

STANDARDS

FOR A

BLOOD TRANSFUSION SERVICE

FIRST EDITION 1958

Prepared jointly by

SCIENTIFIC COMMITTEE OF THE JOINT BLOOD COUNCIL, Inc.

and

STANDARDS COMMITTEE OF THE AMERICAN ASSOCIATION OF BLOOD BANKS

COMPLIMENTARY COPY
The
JOINT BLOOD COUNCIL

Inquiries concerning this publication should be addressed to:

Joint Blood Council, Inc. *Chairman, Scientific Committee* 1832 M Street, N.W. Washington 6, D. C.	**OR**	**American Association of Blood Banks** *Chairman, Standards Committee* 30 North Michigan Avenue Chicago 2, Illinois

Figure 11. The first edition of the AABB Standards, 1958.

is thus to establish procedures that will carry out the intent of the Standards, and then to direct the employees in executing those procedures.

The Technical Manual of the American Association of Blood Banks, on the other hand, is a workbook which suggests procedures which could be adopted to assure that the work of the organizations produces a product of standard quality. The manual procedures are not required but can form the basis for the procedure manual of an organization. Such a procedure manual is an essential part of the property of each blood bank. Each procedure listed in the manual should be reviewed and signed by the director at least annually.

QUALITY ASSURANCE

There is no place for Quality Assurance in the AABB Standards. Like the Ten Commandments, they say what is to be done. They expect quality. Quality Assurance is an Eleventh Commandment. Quality Assurance is necessarily procedural and belongs in the Technical Manual.

But like the first directions of Landsteiner, all our instructions must be brief, simple and clear, in order to assure the quality of the work we direct.

REFERENCES

1. Kendrick, D.B. Blood program in World War II. Washington: Office of the Surgeon General, Dept. of the Army, 1964.
2. International Forum. Does it Make Sense for Blood Transfusion Services to Continue the Time-Honored Syphilis Screening with Cardiolipin Antigen? Vox Sang. 1981;41:183-92.

ADMINISTRATIVE PROCEDURES AND A MACHINE-READABLE SYSTEM TO ASSURE QUALITY CONTROL WITHIN A BLOOD BANK

Z. Smit, H. Smalbil, C.Th. Smit Sibinga

Automation in bloodbanking has involved a variety of approaches, ranging from blood group machine-linked computers to large centralized national systems. The different systems applied show a variety of comprehensiveness and practicability, some being restricted to stock control and issuing of blood, others to filing basic donor information to be used for call-up procedures only. In the USA the Committee for Commonality in Blood Banking Automation CCBBA (1) has made comprehensive information using a barcode principle. Whatever approach or system is used, the main goals of automation are improving safety by preventing and eliminating as optimal as possible clerical errors, thereby providing a usefull tool for assuring the quality of work within the Blood Bank. However, no success will be achieved if one does not start with the fundamental of automation: system analysis.

For administratie and control purposes, we have decided for automation by computer, applying a barcode principle (2,3). Such a computer system needs to be:

a. compact;
b. complete;
c. manageable;
d. terminal connectable.

Automation has been organized primarily for the administrative tasks of:

a. donor administration;
b. laboratory data assimilation;
c. financial administration and invoice;
d. personnel and salary administration, although this part has been put out to contract.

As administration is the objective, the question arises: what does it need to offer? In our philosophy the answer should be:

1. ever readiness – a fast and operational system;
2. accessibility – direct and ready at any time;
3. workload – reduction in workload;
4. cost aspect – cost saving;
5. space problems – space economics of storage and daily operation; and last but not least
6. safety – to prevent administrative and clerical errors.

Based on the above mentioned fundamental considerations we have chosen for an IBM system 34, with 5 terminals, 2 printers, a connected reader-pen for administratie quarantine control and labelling and a reader-pen for issuing the blood.

All donor information is stored in the donor file, consisting of two records per donor (Figures 1a and 1b):
record 1: basic personal information;
record 2: medical information.
The key for every donor is the Restistration Number.

As the Donor Centre deals with over 80 regions, and an efficient mobile team organization, donors are called up in their own region (villages, factories etc.). Therefore the first 2 positions are the region-code, as every region has its own code. The following 6 positions represent the donor's name, where the first 3 positions are a micro-code, deviding the alphabet from 000 till 999, the last 3 positions indicate the sequential number in alphabetical order. A special sub-code can be added, for example '99' is the sub-code for an evening session. When administrating a new donor, the region-code, name and birth date have to be entered and the system automatically provides the micro-code and next sequential number.

DONOR ADMINISTRATION

Record 1	128 digits available	
Registration number	region code	2
	personal	6
	subcode	2
Personalia	sex	1
	name	24
	initials	6
	birth date	7
	street	23
	place	18
	zip code	6
	telephone home	
	area code	5
	number	7
	telephone work	
	area code	5
	number	7
	extension	5
Blood group information	ABO	3
	Rhesus (P/N/U)	1
Total digits used		128

Figure 1a. Donor administration.

Record 2	128 digits available	
Identification (link to record 1)		
registration number	region code	2
	personal	6
personalia	birth date	7
Donation number (last donation)		6
Session information	session date	7
	last response	7
	first donation	7
	last donation	7
	total donations	3
Medical information	Hb	3
	blood pressure	6
	pulse rate	3
	urine	
	albumin	1
	glucose	1
	HB_sAg	1
	syphilis serology	1
	irr. antibodies	9
	ABO	3
	Rhesus phenotype	1
	other blood groups	12
General practitioner		3
Deferral weeks		2
Total digits used		98

Figure 1b. Donor administration.

DONOR CALL-UP PROCEDURE (Figure 2)

When we start a donor call-up procedure, the criteria set by the Donor Centre are entered. The computer searches in the donor data base and makes the selection. Basic criteria for a donor call-up are: region, blood group/Rhesus, period since last donation date. For every session the computer automatically produces:

a. a session list of all selected donors;
b. a label list of these donors, 4 labels for each donor
   1st label – name, adress of the donor
   2nd label – personal information of the donor (to stick on the top of the selection card)
   3rd label – medical information of the donor from two previous donations in code (to stick at the bottom of the selection card)
   4th label – for donor comments;
c. donor call-up cards.

Donor call-up procedure

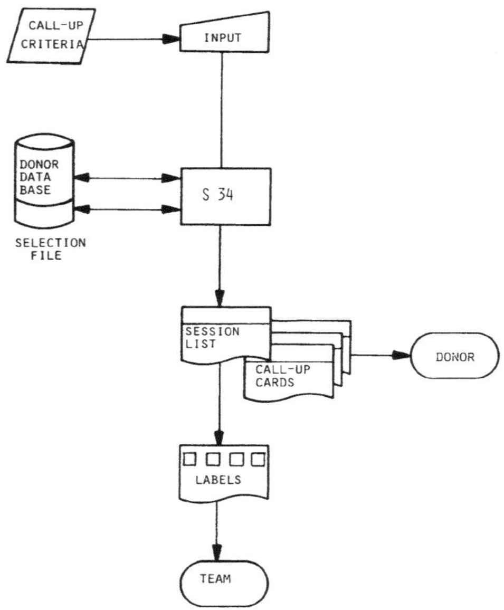

Figure 2

Donor indentification/registration

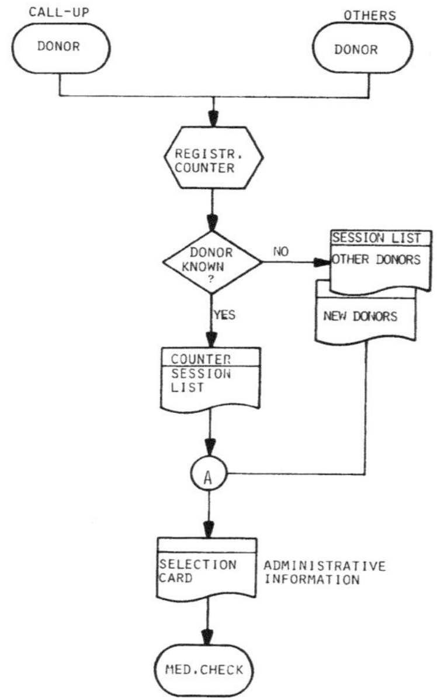

Figure 3

DONOR IDENTIFICATION/REGISTRATION (Figure 3)

During a session we may expect call-up donors, first time donors and spontaneous donors. They are registered at the reception counter. When being known, the donor receives a selection card, labelled with the just mentioned stickers, and can proceed for medical check. When being a first time donor, a selection card has to be written before the donor can go for the medical check. The same procedure can be followed, when a donor is attending the session spontaneously. Now a donor attendant checks the registration number and last donation date from the region check list, prepares the selection card and the donor can go for the medical check.

DONOR SELECTION, MEDICAL CHECK (Figure 4)

With the selection card the donor proceeds to the medical check. When accepted, the donor proceeds to the next step – the donation counter. When not accepted, the donor may be deferred temporarily or definitely. In both cases, after being informed appropriately, the donor goes to the donor canteen for a refreshment.

Donor selection:medical check

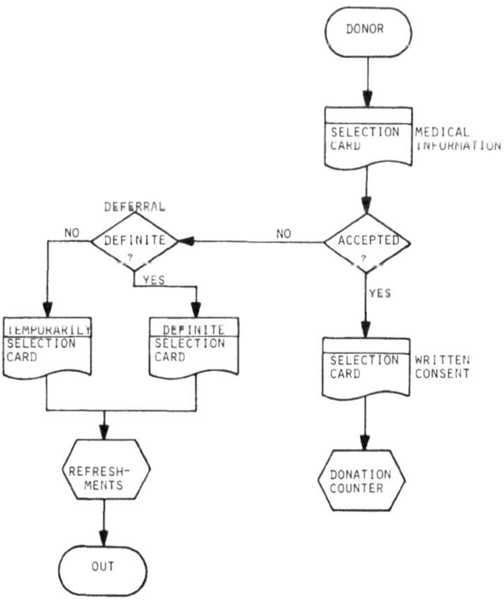

Figure 4

BLOOD DONATION PROCEDURE (Figure 5)

At the donation counter the donor receives a blood bag, pre-labelled with a machine and eye readable donation number. Here, a donor attendant prepares:

1 a list of donation and registration number, being the fundamental of the donation file;
2. a laboratory list.

After having completed the donation, the selection card and the unit of blood are controlled at a seal table. Two pilot tubes are filled out and vertically labelled with the same donation number as present on the blood bag and selection card. These two tubes and the laboratory list go to the laboratory, the filled blood bag goes to the component division and the donor goes to the donor canteen for a refreshment.

Blood donation procedure

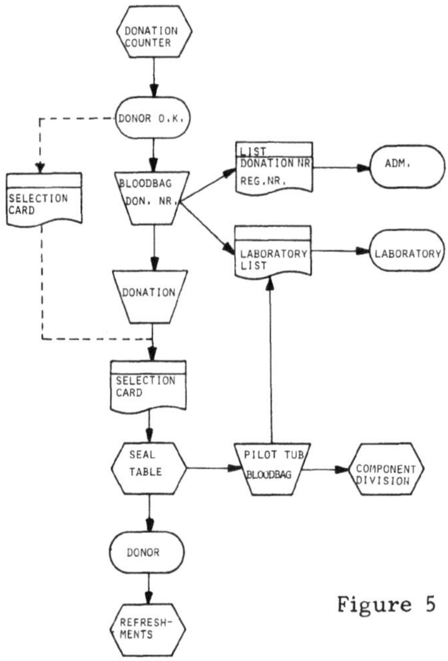

Figure 5

ADMINISTRATION (Figure 6)

The list of donation and registration numbers as produced in the Donor Centre has to be entered in the computer to build up the donation file (Figure 7) and is automatically completed with the blood group/Rhesus of the previous donation from the donor record. First time donors follow in principle the same procedure, but here the blood group/Rhesus information of the previous donation is unknown. The donor record is still empty. A second blood group/Rhesus test is done by control grouping, the result keyed in and automatically compared and matched with the first data (Figure 11b).

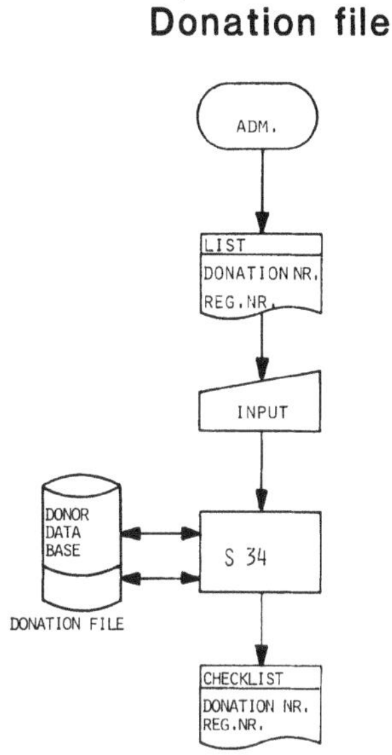

Figure 6

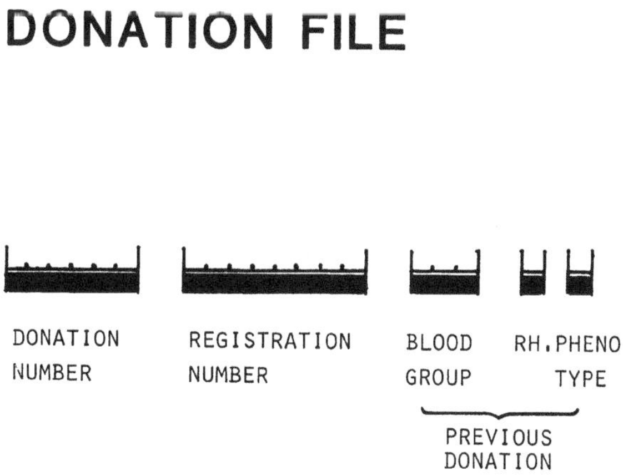

Figure 7

LABORATORY (Figures 8a and 8b)

ABO/Rhesus grouping of donor blood has been automated, using a diskette station connected Technicon BG15, and a connected self designed auto-analyser with a Marsh and Lalezari channel for automated antibody screening. The sampler has been adapted with a moving UV-light source reading device for barcode identification labels (Codabar ®) (4).

The results of all blood group/Rhesus tests are read and decoded in a dataprocessor, stored on a diskette and printed for immediate control (Figure 9). The diskettes are presented to the computer department. The results from hepatitis, syphilis and irregular antibody screening are documented on the original laboratory list. Only the positive results of the test are keyed in individually, the remaining group of negative results are entered "en bloc".

Laboratory administration

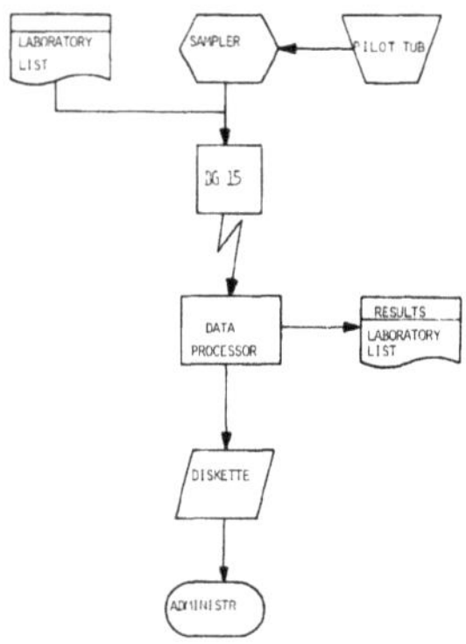

Figure 8a

Input laboratory data

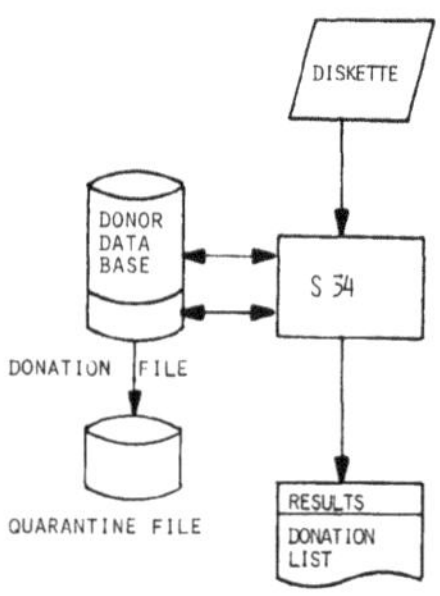

Figure 8b

			===CEL===				==SERUM==				======CEL=======									
list	VLCNR.	M	B	A	A1	AB	A1	A2	B	O	C	c	D	D	E	e	ABO	RHD	AL	
	000000	—	+	+	+	+	—	—	+	—	+	+	+	+	+	+	NTB	NTB.		saline
2104	000000 1	+	-	-	-	-	+	+	+	-	+	+	+	+	-	+	0	POS.		
	000000 2	+	-	-	-	-	+	+	+	-	+	+	+	+	-	+	0	POS.		
	000000 3	+	-	+	-	+	-	-	+	-	+	-	+	+	-	+	A2	POS.		
	000000 4	+	-	+	+	+	-	-	+	-	-	+	-	-	-	+	A1	NEG.		
	000000 5	+	+	+	-	+	-	-	-	-	+	+	+	+	+	+	A2B	POS.		
	000000 6	+	-	-	-	-	+	+	+	-	+	-	+	+	-	+	0	POS.		
	000000 7	+	-	-	-	-	+	+	+	-	+	-	+	+	-	+	0	POS.		
	000033 8	+	+	-	-	+	+	+	-	-	+	+	+	+	+	+	B	POS.		
	000000 9	+	-	+	+	+	-	-	+	-	+	+	+	+	-	+	A1	POS.		
	000000	—	+	+	+	+	—	—	—	—	+	+	+	+	+	+	NTB	NTB.		saline
	000000 10	+	-	+	+	+	-	-	+	-	+	+	+	+	-	+	A1	POS.		
	000000 11	+	-	-	-	-	+	+	+	-	+	+	+	+	+	+	0	POS.		
	000000 12	+	-	+	+	+	-	-	+	-	+	+	+	+	-	+	A1	POS.		
	000000 13	+	-	+	+	+	-	-	+	-	+	-	+	+	-	+	A1	POS.		
	000000 14	+	-	-	-	-	+	+	+	-	-	+	+	+	-	+	0	POS.		
	000000 15	+	+	+	+	+	-	-	-	-	-	+	-	-	-	+	A1B	NEG.		
	000000 16	+	-	+	+	+	-	-	+	-	-	+	-	-	-	+	A1	NEG.		
	000000 17	+	-	-	-	-	+	+	+	-	+	+	+	+	-	+	0	POS.		
	000000 18	+	-	-	-	-	+	+	+	-	+	+	+	+	+	+	0	POS.		
	000000	—	+	+	+	+	—	—	—	—	+	+	+	+	+	+	NTB	NTB.		saline
	000000 19	+	-	+	+	+	-	-	+	-	+	+	+	+	+	+	A1	POS.		
	000000 20	+	-	+	+	+	-	-	+	-	+	+	+	+	-	+	A1	POS.		
	000000 21	+	-	+	+	+	-	-	+	-	-	+	+	+	+	+	A1	POS.		
	000000 22	+	-	+	+	+	-	-	+	-	+	-	+	+	-	+	A1	POS.		
2106	000000 1	+	-	+	-	+	-	-	+	-	+	-	+	+	-	+	A2	POS.		
	000000 2	-	-	+	+	+	-	-	+	-	+	+	+	+	-	+	A1	POS.		
	000000 3	-	-	-	-	-	+	+	+	-	+	+	+	+	+	+	0	POS.		
	000000 4	+	-	+	+	+	-	-	+	-	-	+	+	+	-	+	A1	POS.		
	000000 5	-	-	-	-	-	+	+	+	-	+	+	+	+	-	+	0	POS.		
	000000 6	+	-	+	-	+	-	-	+	-	-	+	+	+	+	+	A1	POS.		
	000000	—	—	+	+	+	—	—	—	—	+	+	+	+	+	—	NTB	NTB.		saline

Figure 9. Automatic readout of the Technicon BG15 machine.
NTB = Niet Te Bepalen (Not interpretable).

LABORATORY DISKETTE (Figure 10)

The laboratory information, ABO and Rhesus, stored on the diskette, is used to build up the quarantine file. The results are printed on a donation list and automatically added to the donation file, completing the so-called quarantine file (Figures 11a and 11b).

LABORATORY DISKETTE

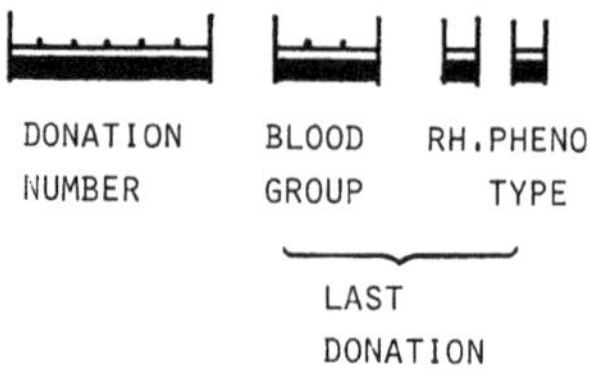

Figure 10

QUARANTINE FILE

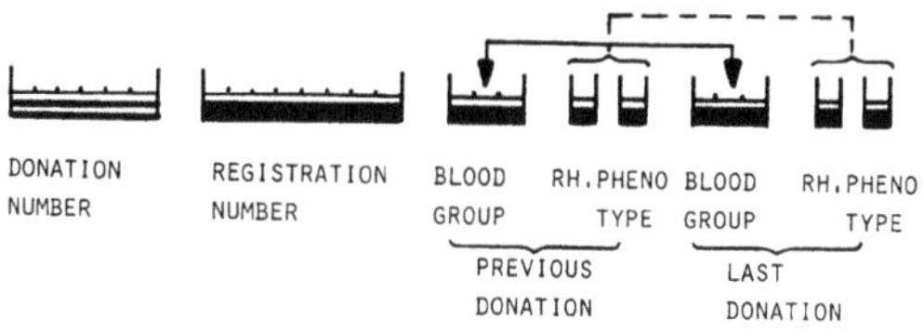

Figure 11a

QUARANTINE FILE : NEW DONOR

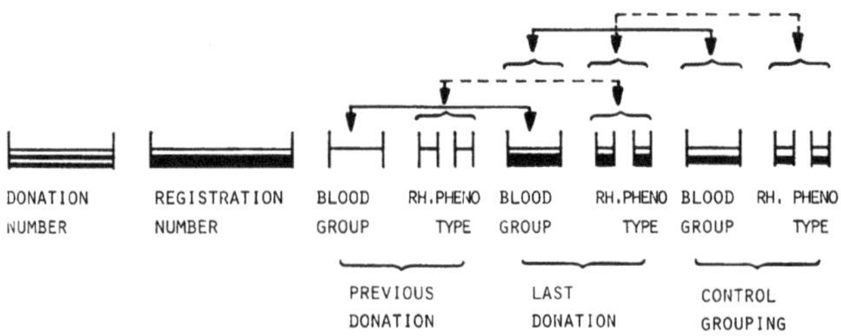

Figure 11b

QUARANTINE CONTROL AND RELEASE (Figure 12)

For labelling the blood bags, the donation number together with the quarantine code, has to be read by reader-pen. The blood group/Rhesus of the previous and last donation are automatically compared in the quarantine file. When blood group/Rhesus are equal, final labelling with a blood group/Rhesus sticker is commanded and for control has to be read again. Then the quarantine file is completed with the product code, resulting in the stock file (Figure 13). When blood group/Rhesus do not match the computer automatically will order to stick a label "hold for further processing" and the laboratory is requested to repeat blood group/Rhesus determination from a tubing sample. All the labelled blood bags have to be counted and the results entered according to blood group/Rhesus. These results are compared with the computer results of the blood bag labelling procedure. Only when the count is correct, the bloodbags can be released to the distribution department.

Quarantine control and release

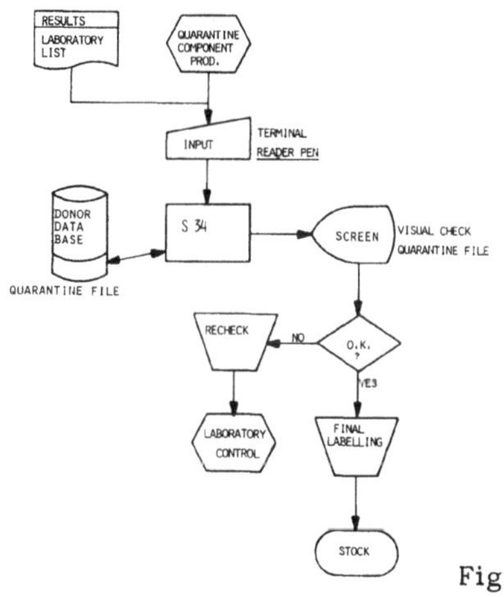

Figure 12

STOCK FILE

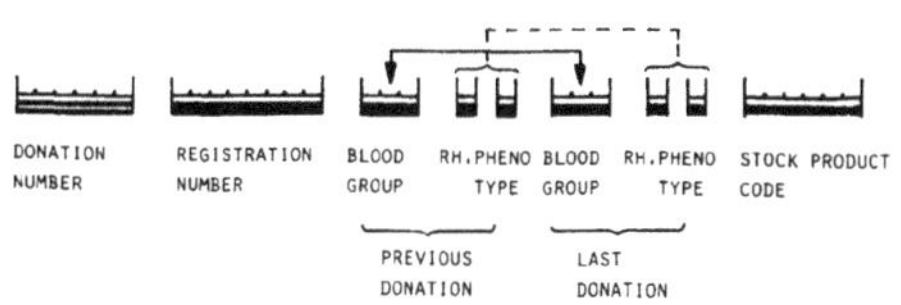

Figure 13

DISTRIBUTION DEPARTMENT (Figure 14)

For practical reasons all 13 hospitals are coded. When a hospital requires blood or blood components, the hospital number or the code is entered and read with the reader-pen. For issuing and billing blood products, the donation number, blood group/Rhesus and product code must be read with the reader-pen for updating the stock file. When the label information is not correct, a piece of tubing is taken from the blood bag for repeat laboratory control and the unit placed back in quarantine. When the label information is correct and the last blood product code has been read, a packing list is produced by a printer, connected with the distribution department terminal. There is always the option to enter data manually instead of reading with a reader-pen. Once a week, the hospitals receive an invoice for all blood products issued.

Administration distribution dept.

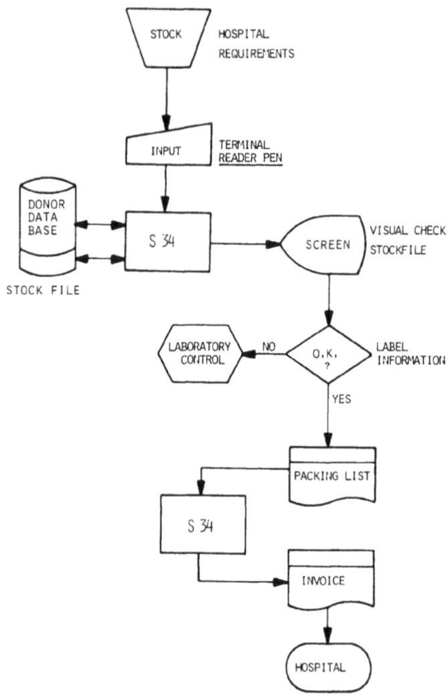

Figure 14

CONCLUSION

The system as it comprehensively covers all practical and administrative aspects in routine bloodbanking from donor to hospital, is now fully implemented in our regional centre. While introducing the system step-wise over the past few years, a surprising and even embarassing amount of clerical errors came to light. It has shown to have a great impact on clerical safety and necessary time commitment of personnel, the keyword being system analysis. Nevertheless, information for the necessary input and construction of the different files has to be gathered, processed and keyed in by human beings. The computer will not tell a lie, unless it has been whispered into its ears – one of the data entering positions. Despite this, the administration procedure as described has proven to be of great impact on clerical safety in the totality of quality assurance within our Blood Bank.

REFERENCES

1. Committee for Communality in Blood Banking Automation. Final Report. Arlington VI, 1977.
2. Bosma, J., Smit Sibinga, C.Th. Automation of a comprehensive Blood Bank administration Transfusion 1979;19:622 (abstract).
3. Smit Sibinga, C.Th., Smit, Z., Smalbil, H., McShine, R.L., de Smit, A.G.J., Waltje, J. A machine readable system for improved quality control in a comprehensive routine Blood Bank. XVII Congress of the ISBT, Budapest 1982. Abstractbook p. 321.
4. McShine, R.L., Das, P.C., Smit Sibinga, C.Th. Continuous automatic recordings of routine ABO and Rhesus bloodgrouping. Transfusion 1979;19:623 (abstract).

QUALITY ASSURANCE OF SEROLOGICAL REAGENTS

W.L. Marsh

The standard of work performed in any laboratory is determined by the expertise of the staff, the availability of equipment and apparatus, and the quality of reagents used. Without high quality reagents the ability of the staff to perform work of high standard is compromised. Probably in no other area of laboratory medicine does the consequence of a mistake have so great a potential danger to the patient as in the blood bank. There is no way in which a clinician can evaluate the accuracy of a blood group report and in this area clinical judgement counts for nothing. It follows that blood group studies, although simple in principle, are heavy in responsibility. Every precaution to ensure accuracy of results must be taken, and a quality assurance program, designed to confirm the effectiveness of reagents before they are used, is an important aspect. Correct handling and storage of reagents is a part of quality assurance, and will be considered in this review.

SALINE SOLUTION

Saline solution, the most widely-used reagent in immunohematology, probably receives the least attention from the viewpoint of quality assurance. Saline contaminated with bacteria may cause non-specific clumping of red cells or, on rare occasions, hemolysis. Contamination with colloidal silica may cause non-specific clumping of red cells, particularly in the anti-globulin test (1). Plasticisers, used during manufacture of plastic containers, may subsequently leach into the contents, and have a detrimental effect on antibody tests. Depending upon the water supply, the pH of water may vary considerably. While mildly acidic water (pH about 6.5) will slightly enhance the results of many red cell agglutination tests, alkaline pH of 9.0 or greater is inhibitory.

In preparing saline solution for use in immunohematology analytical grade sodium chloride should be dissolved in fresh distilled water (ph 6.0 to 7.0) to a concentration of 0.9 gm per cent. The container should be plastic or hard neutral glass, well-washed and rinsed in distilled water to ensure that no residual cleaning agent is present. Heat sterilization of saline solution in soda glass containers is a potential source of contamination with particles of colloidal silica and must be avoided. Do not add preservatives to the saline solution. Continuous "topping-up" of stock saline bottles should also be avoided. When nearing exhaustion, saline containers should be emptied and cleaned before refilling. Saline solutions showing cloudiness or a deposit should be discarded. Any unusual serological results which cast suspicion on the saline should be followed by chemical tests to determine its sodium chloride concentration, a pH test, and by tests for contaminating agents.

BOVINE ALBUMIN

Bovine albumin is widely used in immunohematology to enhance antibody-antigen reactions. The ability to do this depends largely upon the presence of albumin polymers (2). Some albumin preparations cause significant rouleaux formation of red cells, and on rare occasions the reagent may cause hemolysis. New batches of albumin should be tested for these undesirable characteristics. Albumin is used by many workers as a potentiator during the incubation phase of the indirect anti-globulin test. It should be tested by incubation with unsensitized red cells in an indirect anti-globulin test, to confirm that it does not cause false positive results. Albumin contains sodium caprylate, which is added as a stabilizer during manufacture. Rare human sera contain anti-caprylate antibodies which cause agglutination of red cells suspended in stabilized albumin (3). When such "non-specific albumin agglutinins" are encountered, the tests should be repeated omitting albumin from the reaction mixture.

ANTI-GLOBULIN REAGENTS

Anti-human globulin serum, prepared by immunizing animals with human-serum fractions, is one of the most widely used and important serological reagents. The essential characteristics of an acceptable polyspecific reagent are good anti-IgG activity, good anti-complement (anti-C3d) activity and freedom from any tendency to cause non-specific agglutination. In evaluating this reagent it should be tested for its ability to detect a wide range of human IgG blood-group antibodies, and for its ability to agglutinate red cells coated with the C3d component of complement. Anti-globulin reagents are usually diluted to their optimum concentration during manufacture. They should not be further diluted or titrated during evaluation. Anti-globulin serum is the most likely of all blood bank reagents to cause weak false positive results. Negative controls of unsensitized red cells that are included in the evaluation routine should be critically examined.

Most technical errors in bloodbanking are related to performance of the anti-globulin test. The most common mistake is inadequate washing of sensitized red cells, leaving free globulin in the fluid phase. A recommended procedure, which confirms both the effectiveness of the anti-globulin reagent and the thoroughness of the cell washing, is to add weakly IgG-sensitized red cells (e.g. Ortho Coombs Control cell) to one negative test in each batch of anti-globulin tests. This control is particularly important if all tests in the batch are negative.

BLOODGROUP TYPING SERA

The introduction of hybridoma technology into the production of bloodtyping reagents promises a major advance (4). However, in the blood bank reagent field the technique has, as yet, been employed only on a limited scale. Most antisera are still obtained from humans or animals who have been accidentally, or deliberately, immunized. Each individual, or animal, responds to immunization in a slightly different way, and, in most cases, the individual serum contains a heterogenous collection of antibody molecules with slightly different reaction characteristics. It follows that typing reagents which are based on immune sera need careful selection of the serum constituents to ensure acceptable performance and minimum batch-to-batch variation of the finished reagent. Quality assurance thus begins with selection of the reagent constituents, and ends with the day-to-day control procedures employed in the blood bank laboratory.

PRINCIPLES OF QUALITY ASSURANCES

The most important single feature of any testing antiserum is correct specificity. It may be possible to use a reagent with slightly inferior potency, but a powerful reagent that is known to contain a contaminating antibody is unusable.

Three general principles that can be applied to all serological quality assurance routines are:

1. a positive control must always be the most weakly reacting sample that is to be encountered;
2. negative controls, selected to reveal most likely contaminants, are as essential as positive controls;
3. results of control tests should be determined before routine tests are examined.

Applying the first rule, a positive control with anti-A serum, for example, would be an A_2 cell sample. With blood group tests in which antigen dosage is a characteristic of the system, positive controls should always be heterozygous cells. For example, a positive control with anti-Jk^a serum would be a $Jk^{(a+b+)}$ cell sample.

The most likely contaminating antibody in bloodgrouping reagents prepared from human serum is anti-A or anti-B. Although these will be absorbed with appropriate cells, or neutralized with blood group substances, during preparation of the reagent, traces may remain. An A_1 and a B cell sample, that lack the definitive antigen against which the reagent is directed, are included in the quality assurance routine. Specificity, with blood group antisera, cannot be taken to mean absence of all contaminating antibodies. Many antibodies to rare blood group antigens exist and it is not possible during serum selection and reagent preparation to test for, and exclude, all of them. For example about one per cent of random human sera contain anti-Vw (5) although only about 1 in 2,000 people has Vw positive red cells (6,7). It would not be practical to test for, and if present remove, all such antibodies from typing sera, and such sera have a greatly increased incidence of antibodies to rare antigens (8). Many hyperimmune human sera also contain anti-Bg antibodies (9). Presence of anti-Bg in an anti-D serum used for D^u antigen testing by the indirect antiglobulin test, may be a cause of false positive results.

Despite the most stringent precautions in the selection and preparation of blood group antisera, unsuspected contamination with an antibody to a rare blood group antigen is always a possibility. Duplicate tests with different antisera will help detect errors caused by such contaminants but even this precaution is not foolproof. In the case of very rare antisera products of different manufacturers may each be based on serum obtained from the same immunized donor.

All human sera from adults contain polyagglutinins such as anti-T and anti-Tn. They are inevitably present in the immune sera that are used to prepare reagent antisera. Polyagglutinin reactions can usually be recognized by the overall serological behavior of a patient's cell sample. However, the existence of polyagglutinins in nature serve to remind us that most typing sera contain "hidden" antibodies in addition to their specific component.

It is an important principle of quality assurance that the results of control tests should be determined before routine tests are examined. If the results of control tests are unacceptable the routine tests should be discarded without examination, and the tests and controls repeated with fresh reagents. If, despite the warning given by the unacceptable controls, the routine tests are examined and fit with a preconceived idea of the expected results, there is a danger that they will be accepted.

POTENTIATORS

Some antisera contain potentiators such as albumin, polyvinyl pyrrolidone (PVP) or polyethylene glycol (PEG) to promote their agglutinating activity. A side effect of these agents, when present in high concentration, is to induce rouleaux formation of red cells. During initial evaluation of a typing reagent it should be assessed for any tendency to induce excessive rouleaux formation. Strong rouleaux formation may be mistaken for agglutination by an inexperienced worker. Rouleaux formation takes place most readily with red cells of normal discoid shape. Stored red cells slowly assume atypical morphology and are less susceptible to rouleaux formation. The test is made using freshly collected serologically non-reactive red cells, following the recommended test procedure for the reagent. The pattern of red cell distribution is examined microscopically.

STABILITY OF BLOODTYPING REAGENTS

Although justification for routine quality assurance programs include the need to demonstrate acceptable specific activity of a grouping agent, in practice blood group antibodies are relatively stable components of serum and deterioration during in vitro storage is rare. Only if storage conditions are greatly detrimental does the likelihood of loss of specific activity arise. Anti-A, anti-B and anti-Rh_o(D) sera have a great reserve of specific activity, and even with some deterioration would probably still give reliable results. However, rare antisera such as anti-e will have less reserve of potency and any deterioration may have a greater apparent effect. Antisera containing a chemical preservative, such as sodium azide, should be stored in the liquid state at about 4°C. Chemically preserved antisera should not be frozen. Repeated freezing and thawing denatures immunoglobulins and, in addition, produces a local high concentration of antibody and chemical agent in the bottom of the container. Under these conditions deterioration of the antibody may take place more rapidly. Freezing may also affect reagents containing bovine albumin and cause them to give temporary false positive antiglobulin tests (10).

QUALITY ASSURANCE PROTOCOLS

Blood bank reagents are mostly stable preparations, which, when used according to the manufacturers recommended procedure, will give reliable results. The rare discrepancies that occur during usage are invariably caused by accidental contamination or improper storage. The exaggerated day-to-day control routines, that were sometimes advocated a few years ago, can now be seen as expensive, time-consuming, and unnecessary. In the New York Blood Center no example of significant reagent change or deterioration has been detected in routine control tests, during the last 5 years.

The quality assurance procedure has two phases. The first, and most important, is a comprehensive evaluation that determines the specificity, titer, avidity, and stability of new reagents. The second is a simple day-to-day routine that confirms that no deterioration has occurred. As with all ongoing procedures proper record keeping showing control test results are important. These records will allow changes to be traced, should any deterioration of a reagent become apparent. They also serve as a reminder that the tests must be made.

In the initial evaluation of most blood typing sera a titration against appropriate red cells is the only means of comparing the potency of different batches of reagent. Titrations will be influenced by technical variations and by the phenotype of the test cells used. Thus A_2 cells will react less strongly than A_1 cells with anti-A, and R_2R_2 red cells will react more strongly than R_1r red cells when tested with anti-Rh_o(D). In these exercises it is important that all variables should be standardized, in order that results reflect only differences in the reagents themselves. It is good practice to evaluate a number of potential new reagents at the same time. Each reagent should first be transferred to a clean, sterile vial and given a code number. Comparisons will then be objective and not influenced by knowledge of the source. Assessment of a new batch of serological reagent is an important task in a serological laboratory and the test should be made by a skilled technologist.

In day-to-day control routines, one positive and one negative control sample is all that is required. The test is made at the commencement of the day's work and is valid for all subsequent tests made using the same reagent that day. Table I shows control cells that would ideally be used with common antisera.

Table I. Routine control cell samples.

Antiserum	Positive controle	Negative control
anti-A	A_2	B
anti-A_1	A_1	A_2
anti-B	B	A_1
anti-D	O R_1r	A_1B rr
Anti-c	O R_1r	A_1B R_1R_1
anti-C	O r'r (or R_1r)	A_1B R_2r
anti-e	O R_2r	A_1B R_2R_2
anti-E	O r"r (or R_2r)	A_1B rr
Anti-K	O K+k+	A_1B K-k+
anti-Fy^a	O Fy(a+b+)	A_1B Fy(a-b+)
anti-Jk^a	O Jk(a+b+)	A_1B Jk(a-b+)

CONCLUSION

Serological reagents prepared by an experienced and reputable manufacturer are seldom a cause of false results. Errors, when they occur, mostly arise through errors in technique, failure to follow manufacturers recommended procedure, improper storage of the reagent, or use of outdated material. If, during an initial critical evaluation, a reagent is found to be satisfactory it is likely that it will remain so for the period of its dating. Minimal routine control tests are all that are needed thereafter, to confirm that this is so.

REFERENCES

1. Stratton, F., Renton, P.H. Effect of crystalloid solutions prepared in glass bottles on human red cells. Nature 1955;175: 727–8.
2. Jones, J.M., Kekwick, R.A., Goldsmith, K.C.G. Influence of polymers on the efficacy of serum albumin as a potentiator of incomplete Rh agglutinins. Nature 1969;224:510–1.
3. Beck, M.L., Edwards, R.L., Pierce, S.R., Hicklin, B.L., Bayer, W.L. Serologic activity of fatty acid dependent antibodies in albumin-free systems. Transfusion 1976;16:434–6.
4. Kohler, G., Milstein, C. Continuous culture of fused cells secreting antibody of predefined specificity. Nature 1975;256: 495–7.
5. Darnborough, J. Further observations on the Verweyst blood group antigen and antibodies, Vox Sang. 1957;2:362–7.
6. Hart, M.v.d., Bosman, H., Loghem, J.J. van. Two rare human blood group antigens. Vox Sang. 1954;4:108–16.
7. Race, R.R. and Sanger, R. Blood groups in man. 6 ed. Blackwell Scientific Publ. Oxford, 1975, p. 112.
8. Contreras, M., Barbolla, L., Lubenko, A., Armitage, S.E. The incidence of antibodies to low frequency antigens (LFA) in plasmaphersis donors with hyperimmune Rh antisera. Brit. J. Haematol. 1979;41:413–6.
9. Parone, B.G., Issitt, P.D. Anti-Bg antibodies in sera used for red cell typing. Brit. J. Haematol. 1974;27:607–11.
10. Hoppe, P.A.H. Performance criteria for blood grouping sera in: A seminar on performance evaluation. Am. Assoc. of Blood Banks 1976:1–24.

QUALITY CONTROL OF EQUIPMENT

R.E. Klein

It is very difficult to address remarks about quality control testing to an audience of directors and supervisors from a wide spectrum of blood banks and hospital transfusion services. The reason is that some requirements which apply to large donor centers are not applicable to small transfusion services and vice versa. Similarly, the requirements for very large hospital blood banks where patient testing is done many times every day are not the same as for very small hospital blood banks that test only a few patients per week. Since not all aspects can be covered, my remarks will be directed at the medium and small blood banks and transfusion services. Mandatory words will be used, such as "shall" and "must" and advisory words, such as "should". These words are based upon requirements for accreditation of blood banks and hospital transfusion services of the American Association of Blood Banks (AABB). It is not my intent to dictate, but it is necessary to use a foundation for my remarks. If any one at some future date desires AABB accreditation then these remarks will be more meaningful.

The purpose of quality control, as stated in the *Standards for Blood Banks and Transfusion Services* (1) of the AABB, is to ensure that equipment performs as expected. These pieces of equipment must be known factors, because we use these known factors to test donor and patient bloods which are the unknown factors. If the functional capacities of our equipment have not been assured then those also are unknown factors. Then we are testing unknowns with unknowns, and that yields invalid, misleading test results which may result in harm to donors, patients or personnel.

Quality control test methods for equipment must be written in sufficient detail including instructions for personnel actions when test results are inappropriate and entered into the blood bank procedure manual by the medical director. This manual, or a true copy of it, must be available to the technical personnel at all times. All personnel participating in quality control testing must be familiar with the procedures and not deviate in their use. Only in this way will the interpretations of test results be useful and valid, day to day, week to week, month to month, etc.

Functional capacities of most equipment must be assured at four times: (a) upon receipt from the producer or transfer from another laboratory, (b) if in doubt of function during use of the equipment, (c) after repairs or adjustments and (d) periodically during use. Standby equipment also must be tested either periodically while in storage or prior to use for donor or patient testing. It is acceptable for engineering or other service personnel to perform equipment quality control testing but this does not absolve the blood bank director of assuring proper test methods, appropriate results and record preparation and retention. The frequency of testing of equipment while in use is best determined by reviewing past quality control records to determine expected or probable malfunction. But this must not be interpreted that because a piece of equipment has never malfunctioned it does not have to be tested periodically.

THERMOMETERS

Good quality thermometers are necessary for all heat regulated equipment. Mercury in glass thermometers are preferable but cannot be used in freezers which operate below -35°C, because mercury freezes about at -37°C. Good quality electronic thermometers are excellent and can be used for testing freezers. Mercury thermometers should be tested for accuracy upon receipt. Comparing readings of a few thermometers of the same kind at various temperatures within their designated range will reveal those with more than 2°C variations and those should be returned to the distributor. Alternatively, thermometer readings may be compared with a certified, reference thermometer. Subsequent testing of mercury in glass thermometers is rarely if ever necessary. Electronic thermometers should be assured in each range of their intended use at least every six months. Thermometers of alcohol and similar liquids in glass tend to be less accurate expecially when used for a few years.

RH VIEWBOX

The surface of a Rh viewbox must be between 45 and 50°C each day it is used to achieve approximately 37°C of the test mixtures on a glass slide within two minutes. It may require 20 minutes from the time the light is turned on to reach that range. The sensing end of the thermometer should be in contact with the surface of the box for a few minutes before reading. Temperatures near the center and both ends of the surface of the viewbox should be determined about every three months to assure all usable areas are within the acceptable range.

DRY WELL INCUBATORS AND WATER BATHS

For a dry well incubator (heat block), the thermometer should be inserted into a test tube containing a few drops of water. Within a few minutes it must be 35 to 37°C. The test tube with the thermometer should be moved from well to well on initial and annual testings to search for hot or cool wells. If found, these wells should be plugged to preclude use. The thermometer and test tube can then be left in one of the wells for daily quality control readings.

Water baths, both 37°C and 56°C, should each have a thermometer with the bulb end in the water at all times. Temperatures must be of the 35 to 37°C or 54 to 56°C when in use. Upon receipt and then annually, the temperatures near each corner and the middle of the water baths should be measured to assure against hot and cool areas. It is advisable to empty, clean and refill all water baths frequently to control microorganism contamination. This is essential for water baths used to thaw fresh frozen plasma, cryoprecipitate or frozen red blood cells.

If platelet concentrates are stored at 20 to 24°C they must be continuously, gently agitated. This is often referred to as "room temperature" incubation, however, few rooms are maintained continuously at 20 to 24°C. It is the temperature in the immediate vicinity of the platelet concentrates, not at some distant point in the room that must be monitored. A platelet incubator with automatic rotator, heat control and continuous temperature recorder is ideal.

TEMPERATURE RECORDING AND ALARM SYSTEMS FOR REFRIGERATORS AND FREEZERS

Continous temperature recording and an alarm system to warn when temperatures reach undesirable levels are required for equipment in which are stored: (a) whole bloods and blood components and (b) donor and patient blood samples and are strongly recommended for reagents (e.g., antiserums, RRBC's, etc.). Assuring the temperatures of storage for each refrigerator and freezer must be done upon receipt, after repairs and each day of use. The alarm systems must be checked upon receipt and then at monthly intervals.

Each alarm system must either be (a) on a separate house circuit from the refrigerator or freezer or (b) the alarm system must have storage battery power or (c) there must be power failure alarms for the refrigerator or freezer. One of these three is necessary to assure continuous protection of the stored contents. Having the alarm system on an emergency power is not a satisfactory substitute for one of the three named safeguards. Although it is not required, it is highly recommended that refrigerators and freezers be on emergency power. In lieu of emergency power there must be a written procedure for personnel actions to protect the bloods and components.

Temperature recording mechanisms for refrigerators and freezers should be electrical, and at least seven day recorders. The sensor for the recorder must be in liquid in refrigerators but may be in ice in freezers. The container for the liquid or ice must have heat exchange characteristics similar to the container for the donor blood or component being stored. The volume of the liquid or ice should simulate the component of least volume in storage. For example, in refrigerators no more than 250 ml is to be used, simulating the volume of red blood cells. The sensing end of a thermometer is to be in the same container as the sensor of the recorder. Prior to placing the paper disc on the recorder, the date, thermometer reading, personnel initials and identity of the refrigerator or freezer are to be written on the disc where it will not obscure the ink line of the recorder. When the disc is removed, the date, temperature and personnel initials are to be written. Notations are to be written on the disc to explain any ink line beyond the permissible limits. Each day the thermometer reading and the ink line should be compared to assure the ink line is within 1°C of the thermometer and both are between 1 and 6°C.

Alarm systems must be tested at monthly intervals. The sensors of the refrigerator alarm and temperature recorder and bulb end of the thermometer should be places in water at 1 to 6°C and crushed ice added very slowly with stirring. When the alarm sounds, record the mercury thermometer reading. It must be 1.5 ± 0.5°C. The ink line of the recorder should move toward 1°C. Return the sensors and thermometer to water at 1 to 6°C and repeat the above procedure very slowly adding cold tap water (usually 10 to 20°C). Activation of the alarm must be at 5.5 ± 1.5°C. The small up and down deflections on the temperature recording disc should be marked as "monthly alarm test". If there is a remote signal of the alarm system the personnel should respond promptly. The sensors of the recorder and alarm system and thermometer in freezers should be near the door opening opposite the hinges, i.e., the potentially warmest location. To test the alarm system, cover the components, but not the sensors, with a bed blanket or layers of newspapers for an hour or two. Leave the sensors in the container of ice (or liquid). Open the door, read the thermometer and then leave the door open a few centimeters. When the alarm sounds read the thermometer again. Both the first and second readings must be within the acceptable storage temperature. The recorder should have some movement and a notation of "monthly alarm test" is to be written on the disc.

CENTRIFUGES

Upon receipt, if in doubt, after repairs, and periodically during use two perimeters must be assured. The revolutions per minute are best determined with a strobe light. A decrease one test to the next of more than a few hundred RPM is reason to investigate. The timer is to be compared at the interval of use of the centrifuge to include acceleration but not deceleration. If the centrifuge intervals are less than one minute comparison should be with a stopwatch, otherwise any wrist watch or wall clock will do. A variation of more than five seconds per minute is reason to suspect a timer malfunction.

For serologic centrifuges, in addition to the above, a technique for determining the optimum duration of centrifugation is to be used. An acceptable technic and illustration of a record form can be found in Quality Control in Blood Banking (2) by Dr. Byron A. Myhre. The optimum times should be determined upon receipt and after repairs. The interpretations of tests, date and tester's identity should be written on a piece of tape and applied to the centrifuge. These optimum times, for saline (or LISS), cell wahsing and antiglobulin phases must be used for antibody screening of donor and patient blood and crossmatching regardless of the reagent producer's printed directions.

Microhematocrit centrifuges must be assured upon receipt, after repairs and annually for functional capacity of packing donor red cells and every three months for speed and timing. The functional test is to determine the minimum duration (minutes) for maximum packing. Four capillary tubes are three-fourths filled with blood and centrifuged for 3.5 minutes. The packed cell volume (PCV) of each is recorded and the tubes are recentrifuged for 3.5 minutes and the PCV of each is recorded. If no tube shows more than two volumes per cent change after the second centrifugation, then 3.5 minutes is sufficient for use in donor blood testing. Discard the tubes of blood. If any tube showed a two volumes per cent or more change, repeat the test at 4.0 minutes. If 4.0 minutes is not enough then try 4.5 minutes. When the minimum time for complete packing is found, write it, the date and tester's initials on a piece of tape and apply the tape to the centrifuge. The speed and timer tests should be repeated every three months and should not reveal greater than a 15 second variation and no more than a few hundred RPM decline.

Quality control testing of centrifuges used to prepare components consists of temperature determinations, timer and speed verifications and tests of the prepared components. The maximum allowable temperature during the preparation of red blood cells and fresh frozen plasma is 37°C; donor blood from which platelets are to be harvested must be 20 to 24°C; cryoprecipitates must be prepared from plasma between 1 and 6°C. The technique to determine temperatures is simple; at the end of centrifugation, remove two units from the centrifuge, place them back to back (labels facing out), insert the bulb end of a mercury thermometer between the bags and secure the "sandwich" with a rubber band for a few minutes. Assuring the proper speeds is best done with a Strobe light. Tests of the timer are by comparison with a watch or clock. The requirements for quality control of components of donor blood are clearly stated in the Standards for Blood Banks and Transfusion Services of the American Association of Blood Banks.

OTHER EQUIPMENT

Balances used in donor bleeding, to determine the volume of blood drawn, must be tested upon receipt, after repairs and while in use. Each day prior to use the proper location of the metal counter weight should be assured. After completion of the first donor bleeding, weigh the bag but do not include any attached satellite bags. Subtract (a) the weight of the bag and anticoagulant, usually 100 gms, and (b) the weight of any attached, filled, glass pilot tubes. The acceptable range is 430 to 525 gms (equivalent to 405 to 495 ml). Good quality dietary scales, periodically tested with gram weights, must be used.

Rotators for syphillis testing must be assured upon receipt and after repairs for speed and diameter of rotations. If either the speed or diameter is adjustable then it (they) must be assured periodically while in use. Count the rotations for 30 seconds and multiply by two to determine the RPM's. For the VDRL it must be 180 ± 5 RPM per minute and for the RPR 100 ± 2 RPM per minute. Next tape a file card to the platform of the rotator, turn it on and hold a pencil or ballpoint pen against the card to inscribe a few circles. Measure the diameters to ensure 1.8 to 2 cm for VDRL or RPR.

SUMMARY

Quality control testing of equipment is vital in assuring the therapeutic needs of patients and the safety of donors, patients and personnel. Modify or abbreviate when logical the requirements given, do not omit assuring each piece of equipment in your blood bank or transfusion service.

REFERENCES

1. Standards for Blood Banks and Transfusion Services, Tenth Edition 1981, American Association of Blood Banks, Alexandria, VA 22209.
2. Myhre, B.Q. Quality Control in Blood Banking, John Wiley & Sons, NY 1974;106–10.

QUALITY CONTROL OF BLOOD COMPONENTS

C.Th. Smit Sibinga

INTRODUCTION

In assessing definitions, confusion generally starts to grow because of the ever present tendency to ignore the fundamentals and basic philosophies which underlie the defining process. Sir Laurence Peter in his famous Peter Principle (1), analysed the backgrounds of confusion as follows:

1. Many of the experts have actually reached their level of incompetence: their advise is nonsensical or irrelevant.
2. Some of them have sound theories, but are unable to put them into effect.
3. In any event, neither sound, nor unsound proposals can be carried out efficiently, because the machinery of government is a fast series of interlocking hierarchies, ridled through and through with incompetence.

There is much to say for changing of attitude from the rigid and basically nonsensical "quality control", to the more flexible fundamental "quality assurance". Particularly in blood banking, where we deal with a living tissue, a transplant, we have to realise, that in collecting and processing the basic source material, there always will be an element of unpredictability and uncertainty, especially in the final efficacy of the transfusion therapy in clinical medicine.

PRINCIPLES

The principles of quality assurance in blood banking (2) can be defined as:

1. to achieve the desired results;
2. to promote the highest caliber of service to both patient and donor;
3. to minimize the occurrence of problems.

These principles make it possible to set the aims in quality assurance as:

1. to monitor comprehensively the day-to-day service;
2. to analyse problems that will be detected;
3. to initiate appropriate actions to achieve the desired results.

Within the totality of a comprehensive blood transfusion service, a number of variables can be recognized, each with its own importance and impact on the aims of quality assurance:

- there is the donor, the carrier of the raw material: stimulus and motives, selection criteria and desinfection procedures, administrative processes;
- the actual donation: choice of vehiculum (glass vs. PVC) and anticoagulants (heparin, ACD, CPD or CPDA-1), duration and volume of donation;
- processing of each unit taken: time and storage conditions for transportation from donor to component laboratory, processing protocols and conditions, technical support;
- the laboratory control: routine testing (ABO/Rhesus, HBsAg, syphilis and irregular antibodies) and product control (red cell concentrate, platelet concentrate, cryoprecipitate, etc.);
- the storage and issuing: quarantine release procedures, storage conditions and expiration period, conditions for transport to and storage in the hospitals;
- the transfusion practice in the clinic: unique transfusion requirements, giving sets and compatibility of priming fluids, crossmatching;
- the unpredictable response of the patient: final efficacy, improvement of clinical conditions, transfusion reactions.

From this extensive and broad scope of variables, it will be clear that quality assurance needs to be organized carefully and well balanced. Such a program should include and aim for:

1. minimizing donor variations;
2. ensuring maximum detection of in vitro compatibility;
3. assuring administration of the desired type and quality of components for clinical transfusion practice;
4. measuring final in vivo effectiveness in the patient.

Blood transfusion services have been regarded for too long a period of time as institutes of laboratory science combined with milk mans shop type of services. However, the responsibilities of blood transfusion services are twofold and of equal importance:

1. the community, as blood is a national resource, produced, protected and donated by the healthy society, the actual shareholder of the blood bank;
2. the patient, in need of specific components of the blood donated voluntarily and non-remunerated.

The patient finally defines the necessary quality efforts to be put in the organization of blood banks. The organization of a quality assurance program therefore not only comprises equipment, reagents and components, but involves too procedure systems to be used and last but not least the personel. It is the human creature which ultimately does the work and will be responsible for most of the variables and errors. Motivation, teaching and continuous educational exposure and testing are some of the tools in effectively assuring the desired quality of work and guanrantee of final effectiveness of the organization. The extent of quality assurance relates to the type and size of facility, and the amount and diversity of activities in-house as well as related to the society and hospital world. The keystones, however, have te be:

1. manuals, well written and updated;
2. motivation of the personnel, using the manuals in their daily work;
3. continuous education of all workers.

WHO has stated in the 1978 "Requirements for collection, processing and quality control of human blood and blood components", that all criteria of handling and processing should relate to safety, purity, potency and efficacy of any final product to be produced from whole blood or specific collection procedures (3).

The raw material, blood, cells or plasma as given by the donor, need to be processed and controlled optimally, where criteria of safety, purity and potency are of major in vitro importance, assuring the final quality, which will relate to the in vivo efficacy.

More in detail each of these four premises can be described as follows:

1. safety: relates to transmittable disease donor compatibility, sterility, undue toxicity including PKA and hemoglobin;
2. purity: relates to contamination with unwanted cells, proteins, additives, metabolic products from e.g. adenin and other preservatives;
3. potency: relates to expected effectiveness of the product, not only to cell counts or total grams of protein, but more specifically to functional ability or the component, whether this is red cells, Factor VIII or gammaglobulins for intravenous usage;
4. efficacy: the how and to what extent the patient is going to benefit from the transfused final product, and how this relates to storage conditions in the hospital and the ward, the giving sets and priming solutions, contamination at the bed-side, duration of transfusion and co-existing clinical conditions and medication.

Optimal use of human blood therefore depends not only on knowledge, expertise and skill on both sides of the transfusion world – blood transfusion services and clinicians – but depends too on good clinical practice, close co-operation and mutual understanding between blood bankers and clinicians. In the blood bank as a principle each unit taken should be processed into components in the closed multiple blood bag system within 4–6 hours, Factor VIII being the driving force. Whenever necessary and justified each patient should be treated with those components needed to control the clinical situation.

Quality assurance in blood component production can be divided into three main categories:

1. components for immediate clinical use: red cell concentrates and modified whole blood, leucocyte poor red cells, washed red cells and frozen-thawed red cells, platelet concentrates and cryoprecipitate;

2. cytapheresis components: thrombapheresis and leucapheresis concentrates;
3. fractionation source material: fresh frozen plasma, cryosupernatant plasma and out-dated or recovered plasma.

Sample size for quality assurance practice can best be set according to the practice in industry: 1–1.5% of total production. Choice of test systems should be limited to those which provide the desired information and are easily and reproducibly practicable. One must avoid overdoing control for reasons of self-satisfaction. Blood banks must not develop into quality control laboratories, without contact with clinical reality!

PRACTICE

In our regional Red Cross Blood Bank, covering a 1.1 million population and serving 13 hospitals or 5000 acute beds on an annual donation rate of 50,000/million population, bloodtransfusion is practiced on an all component basis. Quality assurance is organized in a practical way with an immediate responsibility to the bed-side situation where the blood and the components are used to treat and support the patients.

For each division there are protocolled in-process quality assurance procedures, whether Donor Centre, Administration, Laboratory or Component Division. The laboratory, being the division for routine and product quality control, is responsible for testing the samples from donors, collected blood or component produced. There too is a task in testing samples derived from patients and units of components involved in transfusion reactions. Results are discussed on a weekly basis, and statistics are presented in a monthly staff meeting. In-process control for each individual component comprises tests for qualitative and functional aspects, relating to the ultimate clinical use.

The following schemes show the basic in-process program for the different components:

Table I. Red cell products.

Product	Test	Frequency
Whole blood (processed, expired)	a. weight b. sterility c. pinholes	monthly weekly dayly
Red cell concentrate (expired)	a. hematocrit b. sterility	monthly weekly

Table II. Leucocyte poor blood.

Product	Test	Frequency
Leucocyte-poor rcc	a. leucocyte count pre-filtration and post-filtration	monthly
	b. hematocrit	monthly
	c. sterility	weekly

Table III. Platelet concentrate.

Product	Test	Frequency
Platelet concentrate (expired)	a. weight	monthly
	b. pH	monthly
	c. platelet count	monthly
	d. sterility	weekly
	e. platelet function	optional

Table IV. Cryoprecipitate.

Product	Test	Frequency
Cryoprecipitate	a. weight	monthly
	b. Factor VIII:C	monthly
	c. alloagglutinins	monthly
	d. sterility	weekly
	e. fibrinogen	optional
	f. total protein	optional

Table V. Plasma products.

Product	Test	Frequency
Fresh frozen plasma	a. weight	monthly
	b. Factor VIII:C	monthly
	c. sterility	weekly
	d. albumin	optional
	e. total protein	optional
Single donor plasma (cryosupernatant)	a. weight	monthly
	b. sterility	weekly
	c. albumin	optional
	d. total protein	optional

CONCLUSION

Quality assurance is of extreme importance, particularly in blood-transfusion where we deal with a delicate and precious material, human blood – a living tissue.

When we agree on the principles and the fundamentals of the organization and ultimate aims, we will conclude that the most unpredictable variable in the system is the human being, who does the job.

Motivation, continuous education and above all dedication to both donor and recipient, taking full responsibility for the handling, processing, storage and transfusion of the "gift of life", are undoubtedly the main tools for a successful program of assuring quality of blood components.

REFERENCES

1. Peter, L.J., Hull, R. The Peter Principle, Toronto/New York/ London, Bantam books, 1969.
2. Taswell, H.F., Saeed, S.M. Principles and Practice of Quality Control in the Blood Bank, Washington DC: American Association of Blood Banks 1980.
3. World Health Organization. Technical Report Series 626, Geneva 1978.

IMMUNOGLOBULIN PRODUCTION: ORGANIZATION AND QUALITY CONTROL OF SOURCE MATERIAL

R.J. Crawford

In the United Kingdom the terms quality assurance and quality control have special meanings:

Quality assurance is a total system of organized working (and testing) designed to ensure the quality of products.

Quality control consists of tests which must be completed with satisfactory results before a donation or a batch of product may be issued. Quality control is a part of quality assurance.

Following on from these definitions, the system of working first and the tests later shall be described.

The collection of plasma for specific immunoglobulin preparation is a complex undertaking and it is impossible to describe it simply. In describing our system, the places where mistakes can be made, and where they can be prevented will become clear. The purpose is to allow the reader to apply the philosophy of quality assurance to his own circumstances in his own center.

DONOR SELECTION

There are three approaches to donor selection. One can select a target group of people with a high prevalence of the required antibody, one can screen existing donors or one can recruit volunteers for boosting. Plasma may then be harvested from whole blood donations or by plasmapheresis. This choice is discussed later.

Let us look in detail at screening target groups as it is the most complicated method. We have arrangements with family doctors who notify cases of infectious disease in fit adults. This is a major source of antizoster donors. In Scotland the virus laboratories all report positive results to the Communicable Diseases Scotland, a unit which publishes the age, sex, diagnosis and laboratory findings in its weekly journal. When we find a report of an antibody which we need, the virologist puts us in touch with the clinician in charge of the patient. He is the final judge of whether we may attempt to recruit his patient.

Another method is to follow up vaccinations. Rabies vaccine is used by a very small number of doctors and they tell us about their cases. For some reason we have much less success with smallpox and diphtheria vaccinees. Both of these vaccines are still occasionally used among staff of infectious diseases units. Vaccines against chickenpox, CMV and botulism are not used in Scotland. Some regions keep central records of vaccinations, for instance, colleagues in Inverness get details of possible anti-tetanus donors from the public health computer.

It is necessary to ensure that target populations are validly selected. We found that 24% of a group of workers given regular tetanus toxoid were hyperimmune compared with only 5% of ordinary donors. On the other hand our study of people in contact with cases of chickenpox showed that this was not a useful source of high titre donors.

PLASMA COLLECTION

There are two methods of collecting antibody: donors may be plasmapheresed or plasma can be taken from whole blood donations. Each has its advantages and disadvantages and skill is required to find the ideal combination in a given set of circumstances.

Plasmapheresis is most useful for uncommon antibodies where donors are hard to find or for antibodies where long term mass screening is prohibitively expensive. Generally plasmapheresis is only applicable to antibodies where high titres persist for months or years, though even within a single antibody specificity there is considerable variation between donors. Unfortunately not all donors are able to give up time for frequent visits to the donor center and travelling expenses are high. In our region we do plasmapheresis at two centers 37 km apart and we recently had to transport two donors from the same town one to each center. As appointments are made to suit the donors and are often changed at short notice efficient transport arrangements are almost impossible to organize.

If you have the good fortune to find donors who have recently been immunized or boosted one can plasmapherese intensively for a few months, then rest the donor. In this way one can collect good quantities of antibody even if each donor only maintains his titre for a few weeks.

With most antibodies you need to be alert to falling titres and remove the donors from the plasmapheresis program. In the summer of 1981 one third of all our anti-tetanus plasmapheresis procedures yielded plasma with unsuitable antibody levels. The main cause was donors whose antibody levels had fallen between the initial screening and the first plasmapheresis appointment available. Therefore the panel must be refined continuously. Donors whose titres have fallen must be replaced by new ones until the plasmapheresis panel consists largely of donors with chronic high titre antibody. If this policy is not vigorously enforced the staff become so friendly with the donors that they insist on continuing to collect what is really only normal plasma. The program then becomes full and there is no space for new donors.

The other way to obtain plasma is to collect whole blood. The red cells are then available for transfusion. Our current estimate is that it actually costs more to collect plasma this way unless the red cells are required for the blood bank.

Harvesting of antibody containing plasma from whole blood is only practicable if a high proportion of blood is collected in multiple packs and processed to fresh frozen plasma in individual unpooled donations. Obviously the donations have to be kept until screening results are available.

The whole blood method works best when 3 or 5 per cent of donors have useful titres and either the screening test is cheap or titres fall rapidly. You can obtain plasma from donors who give blood at mobile sessions distant from your plasmapheresis centers. Another advantage is that one does not need an elaborate appointment system, the donors are called by the computer in the normal way.

Apart from getting the plasma there are two options for future collections (a) switching the donor to plasmapheresis or (b) putting a flag on his computer record to remind that his next donation will be worth screening.

CONTROL OF PLASMA

The actual quality control is not easy. A moderate sized transfusion center processes 500–800 donations of plasma per day. The demand for anti-tetanus and anti-hepatitis requires nearly 100% screening for each. In addition a smaller number of donations needs to be screened for CMV, rubella, varicella-zoster and so on. The last three are done for us by an outside laboratory and the results take a day or two to become available.

Plasmapheresis donations are collected with a particular antibody in mind. They come to the center labelled with the name of the antibody and there is a constant risk that these donations will be put directly into stock instead of being quarantined until the antibody level has been checked.

We now have a separate department which determines the fate of plasma donations. It works independently of the main processing department. It does not matter whether your quarantine is physical or computer based or just written on work sheets but it is essential to have a responsible person in charge who will devise a good system and operate it conscientiously.

ANTIBODY ASSAYS

The assays chosen should be inexpensive and should be sufficiently simple and robust to allow large numbers of tests to be done by the staff available. Not all antibody produced to an immunogen is biologically significant and it is important that the assay chosen should reflect the concentration of <u>protective</u> antibody. For this reason assays should be calibrated against biological neutralisation assays wherever possible. The assay method used should give a linear dose-response performance at the antibody concentration required by the fractionation center. I do not know of any assay which conforms fully to these criteria. The following examples will illustrate the problems.

Anti-tetanus is assayed in our center by counter immuno electrophoresis for screening and by RIA for clinical work. Elsewhere in Scotland immunodiffusion haemagglutination and EIA are used. Individually each gives acceptable correlation with mouse protection although the EIA gives inaccurately high results with very strong antibodies. Seven plasmas and a well calibrated working standard were used to prepare a proficiency test of 20 specimens. A consensus was obtainable on only 17, but each test was generally close to the consensus on most specimens. RID gave false high results in 3 tests (including the same material twice, so this represented two specimens). CIEP gave two low results and HA gave two high results on the same sample but unfortunately owing to the cut off of the test there was a number of results whose agreement or otherwise with the consensus could not be determined. Thus, in general each test gave good results but there were exceptions.

There is a possibility that results on some sera are repeatably inaccurate by a particular technique. The only way to deal with this is to calibrate tests using very large numbers of sera of known neutralising antibody content. Unfortunately the neutralisation test is both expensive and imprecise so large surveys are not practicable.

Our CIEP test always detects the 10 IU/ml control and never the 5 IU/ml low control, but further examination is required to ensure that the cut off is not fluctuating in the 5–10 IU/ml range.

When a large number of donations is being tested imprecision has a limited effect on overall antibody yields but when donors are being called for plasmapheresis and then being removed from the program good precision is essential.

We chose CIEP because it works well in our hands and we have all the equipment, because we used CIEP for hepatitis B surface antigen screening until 1974. CIEP is not so quantitative as immunodiffusion but is quicker and easier to read. It is cheaper than haemagglutination and does not require sample dilution and processing equipment like EIA.

Antibody to hepatitis B can also be tested by CIEP, but the test is less precise than it is for anti-tetanus. Some laboratories use haemagglutination but this involves expensive reagents as few centers still coat cells with HBsAg or anti-HBs. We use an RIA based on reuse of labelled anti-HBs from negative Ausria II tests. The recovered antibody is pooled and each batch is subjected to quality control before use. The test is a solid phase inhibition RIA and is a little over-sensitive to avoid failing to detect useful antibodies. All the positives are reassayed to indentify those above 10 IU/ml.

We are currently using CIEP, but are hoping to devise a semi-quantative RIA – diluting samples to put them on to the linear part of the dose response curve.

Work load considerations are important. Our microbiology laboratory tests all donations for HBsAg by RIA, most for anti-tetanus by CIEP and most for anti-HBs by RIA. All initial screens are completed the working day after collection. In addition ante-natal sera are screened for HBsAg by low-cost RIA as part of the vertical transmission program. The next development should be to introduce a CMV screen to provide CMV negative products and high titre plasma for immunoglobulin.

To return to the theme of this conference: Quality assurance is a total system of organized working ... We have still a long way to go.

BACTERIAL SURVEYANCE IN A BLOOD BANK

P.C. Das, C.Th. Smit Sibinga, J. Dankert

INTRODUCTION

Bacterial contamination of blood, causing injury to patients, is phylosophically an anethema, since blood is supposed to save lives – not to cause injury. As any infusion fluid, the potential risk of contamination from blood does exist, especially since blood and its products are themselves good growth media.

During the last decade several such accidents have been reported (1), but the sterile closed plastic system has significantly minimised this risk (2). On the other hand, the intensity of handling and processing of a single unit of blood has increased the risk of contamination; some products such as red blood cell concentrates are left in storage with virtually none of the plasma that traditionally provides an anti-bacterial defence medium. Thus, the potential for bacterial growth may have increased. The traditional visual criteria for checking bacterial contamination is difficult to apply in the plastic bag system with different blood products. However, blood transfusion services regularly undertake bacterial sterility control studies when a product becomes "open" or when blood and its products are implicated in transfusion reactions.

During the "50s" prospective studies were carried out in relation to bacterial contamination (3,4); but presently little has been done to measure bacterial incidence prospectively to quantify and measure the sites of importance in the processing chain.

THE AIM AND DESIGN OF THE STUDY

This work was designed to investigate the potential risk and the source of bacterial contamination of blood and its components at the time of collection at the donor side, during the handling and production of components and its storage in the blood bank, and the point of transfusion at the patient's bed-side.

BLOOD DONATION

Accepting the manufacturer's guarantee of sterility of the closed plastic bag system we concentrated on the withdrawal procedure from the donor. Proper cleaning of the skin with chlorohexidine in alcohol for 10–20 seconds would ensure disappearance of transient flora during and untill the end of the donation. This is shown in Figure 1 where a longitudinal culture study was carried out on samples from donor skin to evaluate the effects of skin desinfection. Phlebotomists' fingers are also a potential source of bacteria. Desinfection of fingers at regular 15 minutes intervals is not sufficient, since recontamination can occur within 5 minutes. Thus, each venepuncture should be preceded immediately by decontamination of the hand.

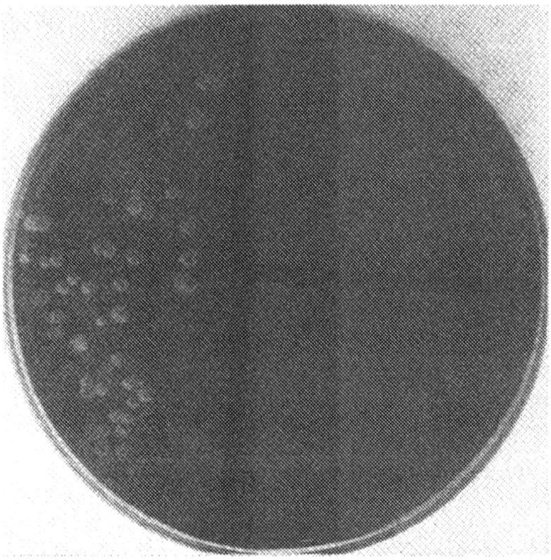

Figure 1. Results of desinfection procedure on donor skin. Left: predesinfection growth in colonies. Upper right: immediately after desinfection. Lower right: immediateley after donation.

Table I. Materials tested over 2 periods.

	1977			1980		
Item studied	total	growth	%	total	growth	%
Cellular component	305	8	(2.6)	480	10	(2.0)
Plasma component	107	3	(2.3)	174	2	(1.1)
waterbath	28	18	(64.3)	64	0	(0)

Table II. Bacteriological control over 1980 – isolated microorganisms.*

		Streptococcus species	Bacillus species	Flavo bacteria	Staphylococcus citicus	Streptococcus viridans	Acineto bacterie species	Staphylococcus epidermidis	
Whole blood	142	1	3					1	
rbc	129		1						
Leuc. poor rbc	79							1	
Platelet concentration	130							3	
S.d. plasma	75								
Cryoprecipitate	27								
Fresh frozen plasma	20								
Outdated plasma container	52							2	
Waterbath	64								
	728	1	4					7	12 positive
* for 1981	832		7					3	10 positive

PRODUCTION OF BLOOD AND ITS COMPONENTS

Potential bacterial contamination at this stage was investigated by studying:

1. collection bags;
2. the bacterial control of immediate environments e.g. waterbath;
3. cultures of individual products: both cellular and plasma components taken randomly after appropriate storage. The sample size was about 1–2% of the total product.

Over the last 5 years no pinhole was seen in the bags. During this period we carried out bacterial culture on different products. The results of 1977 and 1980 (Table I) are presented for comparison. Our initial problem was related to a waterbath contaminated with Pseudomonas species and E. coli. The demineralised water supply was partly responsable for the organisms. With a proper water supply, regular cleaning and an especially made desinfectant (chlorohexidine in NaN_3), this problem appears to have been almost eliminated. Contamination may be due to sampling techniques or to environmental contamination during sampling (1.1–2.6%) but the majority of contamination is skin commensal organisms (Table II). If some of the positive cultures were derived from blood and its products, this would indeed support the earlier finding of 1–4% positive cultures reported in the literature (5,6).

AT THE BED-SIDE

Any untoward reaction in a patient due to transfusion of blood or its products was encouraged to be reported. Investigations of routine transfusion reaction procedures are followed, and a sample from the offending products was sent for bacteriological culture. Three years cumulative data are presented in Table III. As a contrast, the total number appropriate of products delivered during this period is also presented. Since our blood bank serves 5000 acute beds in 13 hospitals, the under-reporting of transfusion associated reactions seem to be the norm. For example, only 4 units of leucocyte poor blood were implicated out of the total of over 20,000 such products used. However, the incidences reported reflect a cross section of the proportional use of the different products in our region (cryoprecipitate excepted).

In interpreting these results the following aspects need to be considered. Mostly the materials are returned in an opened system, sometimes having been kept at room temperature. The length of time elapsing between a reported transfusion reaction and the request for investigation can vary from 2– 7 days. Furthermore, when a closed "pigtail" attached to the mother bag was available for examination, the positive culture could not in all cases be substantiated. This implies technical sampling problems during bacterial culturing or environmental problems in hospital wards.

At the transfusion site the same aseptic techniques such as described in the blood withdrawal section should essentially be followed, but this "art" can vary depending on urgency, staff load, weekend and other factors. We have been known to follow

Table III. Results of bacteriological investigation of blood and blood components involved in transfusion related reactions (1979–1981).

Aliquot	total transfusions	total	with growth	Gram pos	Gram neg	fungi
Whole blood	43,465	33	2	+	-	-
rcc	62,609	133	5	+	-	-
Leucocyte poor blood	20,107	4	1	+	-	-
Platelet concentrate	14,501	2	-	-	-	-
Cryoprecipitate	56,969	5	-	-	-	-
Total	197,651	177	8	+	-	-

the trail of a product over tables and into corners of wards "en route" to the patient. The results show (Table IV) that there is a fairly even chance that blood and its products can accidently and inadvertantly be contaminated even at the side of an operation. When the patient's vascular access is difficult, the infusion set usually remains in place and is used for various other intravenous infusion fluids and possibly medicaments. In this situation it is unreasonable to expect the resident to send the infusion set for investigation. Thus, important information for this type of study is lost.

Table IV. Bacteriological investigation in hospital wards.*

Item studied	growth/ml
Cryo waterbath	10^3 Bacillus species < 10 Staphylococcus epidermidis
Glassfibroscope	< 10 Staphylococcus epidermidis
Waterbath (ward)	Pseudomonas species

* Study over a month, only positive results reported.

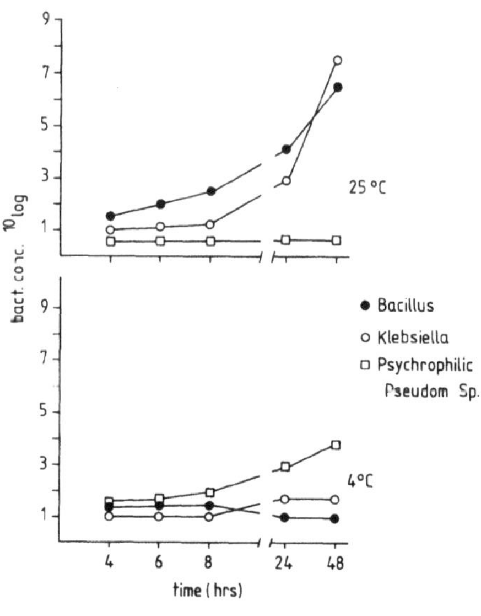

Figure 2. Rate of multiplication of 3 bacterial species in packed cells at 4°C and 25°C.

There are microorganisms capable to grow at low temperatures called psychrophilic bacteria. Sometimes they may cause problems. At room temperature, they as well as other inadvertantly introduced organisms, show an increased rate of growth, and therefore become detectable (Figure 2).

CONCLUSION

This study re-emphasizes the fact that bacterial contamination of blood is not yet archaic. The considerable handling a unit of blood undergoes during processing, should be contrasted with the (false) sense of security brought about by use of the closed plastic bag system. Strict asepsis and antiseptic protocols are still important at all stages.

Environmental contamination probably plays an important role especially at the patients' bed-side about which little information is available. The dramatic endotoxic shock following Gram negative contamination is well recognized (7). But one should remember that while non-pathogenic commensal organisms may be technical artefacts in this study (8), they can cause ill effects in immunosuppressed leukemic and oncology patients. Blood banks should be encouraged to follow the lead of the pharmaceutical industry in the quality of bacterial surveillance of their products; this study by no means tries to claim anything of that order. But it illustrates an attempt to follow an old adage – the better the devil you know than the devil you do not know.

ACKNOWLEDGMENTS

M. Lamers and M. Knippers contributed to this project as a part of their university study in the Faculty of Pharmacy. We are grateful to Dr. J.A.M. Snijder for his interest and also undertaking some of the bacterial investigations at the Public Health Laboratory, Groningen.

Anje Luchtenberg has typed many drafts of this presentation.

REFERENCES

1. Telegraaf (Dutch daily, Amsterdam), September 8, 1979.
2. Honing, C.L., Bove J.R. Transfusion associated fatalities: review of Bureau of Biologies Report. Transfusion 1980;20:653–61.
3. Geller, P., Jawetz, E. Experimental studies on bacterial contamination of bank blood. J. Lab. and Clin. Med., 1954;43:696–706.
4. Pittman, M. A study of bacteria implicated in transfusion reaction and of bacteria isolated from blood products. J. Lab. and Clin. Med., 1953;42:273–88.
5. Cordle, D., Koepke, J.A., Koontz. The sterility of platelet and granulocyte concentrates. Transfusion 1980;20:105–7.

6. Wrenn, H.E., Speicher, C.E. Platelet concentrates sterility of 400 single units stored at room temperature. Transfusion 1974;14:171–2.
7. Brand, A.I. Transfusion reaction from contaminated blood. N. Eng. J. Med. 1958;258:1289–93.
8. Walter, C.W., Koudsin, R.B., Balton, L.N. New technique for detection of bacterial contamination in a blood bank using plastic equipment. N. Eng. J. Med 1957;257:364–9

DISCUSSION

Moderators: P.C. Das, B.A. Myhre

W.L. Marsh, New York, USA:

Could I make a remark related to Mr. Smit's observations on automation? It is very important we should remember that the mere introduction of automation does not mean we do not need quality control. There are assumptions some people seem to make that the machine will not make mistakes. This is quite untrue. I think it is very important in alternative routine, to have strict quality assurance. The machine cannot think, but we can. When we are evaluating routines and evaluating results, we can look at it subjectively and make decisions.

I would like to point out that the quality assurance needed is really quite extensive. We have three Groupamatics to type the donors, and extensive quality assurance routines on the automated process itself. For example, when you are feeding samples through a sample identification, there is always the possibility that the machine will go out of synchronization. So, one certainly has to think very carefully how to set this up. It is not sufficient, for example, simply to put every 20th or every 50th sample as a negative or positive.

It is also very important on computer routines of this kind that all the surveillance must be done by the computer itself. The acceptance of the quality control procedures in a computer routine should not be made by the individual, it must be made by the computer. I think these are the points which are important.

P.C. Das, Groningen, The Netherlands:

Could I call on Dr. Smit Sibinga to take up the point which Dr. Marsh made.

C.Th. Smit Sibinga, Groningen, The Netherlands:

There is a real potential danger the moment you start using machines and automation, because we all know that many of us regard these machines as the most reliable equipment we have. What we frequently come across is that technicians go for a cup of coffee, leaving the blood group machine to its own devices.

This is a wrong attitude. The moment we use computers, the mistakes can be greater in quantity and in quality. For instance, at the blood bag issuing counter in the Donor Center the most important information is collected, on which we rely for converting the information on the donation number together with the registration number of the donor. When in the necessary transcription a mistake is made, the chain of events goes right from the Blood Bank to the patient. It leads to the realization that an error has been made: what is in the bag, is not what the donor has given. We should be well aware of the fact, that those who have to key in information should be very skilled and very allert in their job.

B.A. Myhre, Torrance, USA:

A very brief question. How often do you back up your records? How do you check to make sure that you have not lost some of the data that you are going to back up?

C.Th. Smit Sibinga:

We back up the records every day. There is a print-out made for control to see that we have keyed in correctly our information to back up the records.

R.J. Crawford, Glasgow, Scotland:

We have got a computer system which uses a somewhat different donor registration system number. How can we go from the name and date of birth of an individual to a six-digit registration number? If I told you my name and date of birth, could you tell me what my registration number would be at Groningen-Drenthe?

The second question: If for example I was an established donor in one part of your region, and I moved to another part of the region, I would still have the same number, but would it only be my place of donation number that would change?

Z. Smit, Groningen, The Netherlands:

Given a name and date of birth, our computer is able to trace the registration number of the donor. When a donor moves to another area in our region, he carries the same registration number, which is the last 6 digits, but the area code number would change, which is the first 2 digits of the number. Of course, donation number is different.

W.L. Marsh:

Let us continue the discussion we had earlier: the importance of identification.

We have to realize that there are some errors and so we need to have some working safeguards. The safeguards we use, for example, in New York concern laser scanner reports and the computer that surveys them. Only three identical readings by the scanner will be accepted by the computer. If three readings are not identical, then the computer will not accept the entry. I think it is important to realize that errors may occur and we have to build in a system to make sure to try and avoid them when we can.

Th.M. Brouwers, Deventer, The Netherlands:

Dr. Das do you have routine bacteriological control of certain products in your Blood Bank? What are the arguments for it in a statistical context?

P.C. Das:

The answer is yes. The idea occurred to me that the devil that you know is better than the devil that you do not know. That is the philosophy we adopted when I started five years ago. It is quite clear that we see two approaches in component production. One is the pharmaceutical industry which applies very stringent rules and the other is the Blood Bank which is less stringent. We should try to move to a higher level, in order to achieve that we should determine what the problem is at the Blood Bank level. This vital information we tried to collect over five years from three sources related to blood collection, processing and to the patients' bed-side. I have tried to show that bacteriological problems in these areas, although minor, still exist.

P. Rebulla, Milan, Italy:

One should try to decide when to do quality control during storage of a particular blood component. To me, this applies in particular to a delicat component such as platelet concentrate. Although the platelet concentrate expiration time is a point under discussion, we think that "the fresher, the better". In our institution we follow the "last in-first out" policy, which allows us to transfuse 70% of patients with fresh ($\leq$ 24 hr of collection) platelet concentrates. For this reason we carry out the quality control program (platelet count, pH, and temperature of storage) on platelet concentrates stored for 24 hr, and not after 72 hr of storage or immediately after production.

C.Th. Smit Sibinga:

There are several options open. We have chosen for platelets at the end of shelf-life – looking at the number of platelets still "countable", looking at the pH as a condition for preservation, for keeping the platelets in good order and for conducting tests on the hemostatic capacity. Why do we choose expired platelets? Because platelets are so valuable that we do not like to involve platelets which we need, at that particular point of quality control. When platelets are at the 72-hour limit – which is a deadline – and if they are still in good order, one can be sure that when going back up the line to the point of collection, they will be good as well; the 72 hours is an optional point. We have done tests up till the 72 and the 120 hours deterioration starts. There are new developments on the horizon. In the USA already in application, new plastics, PVCs with a different type of plasticiser (trimeliate instead of DEHP), as well as polyolefine, show clearly that one can keep platelets up to at least 120 hours for clinical use with adequate hemostatic capacity.

P.C. Das:

Could I direct a question to Dr. Crawford? When I came to the Continent from Scotland, I planned to collect plasma with antibodies against viruses, tetanus and others for eventual immunoglobulin fractionation. It was, however, pointed out to me that these specific immunoglobulins were not so in demand on the Continent. Could you tell me why there is such a difference of practice between the UK and the Continent?

R.J. Crawford:

I do not know how many of you know that the smallest exposure to any hepatitis B-containing material is 30% lethal. Our newspapers in Scotland seem to know that! We are working against a perspective of the most terrible fear of hepatitis B. This is why so much anti-hepatitis B immunoglobulin is used. I recently saw a paper from the USA which reports the staff incidence of hepatitis B among health-care personnel is some per cent per annum. We count per hundred thousand per annum. Mind you, our figures are slightly higher. So, I am not saying it is a thousand times less common, but we set our brains three orders of magnitude lower, and there still is a panic in Scotland.

As for anti-tetanus, there is one Glasgow hospital which uses more than 50% of Scotland's national uptake of anti-tetanus immunoglobulin. There are beautiful criteria set up by the British Government on how to use it, but they have woollt things like a "significant wound". These people think almost all wounds are a high risk for tetanus because the skin has been broken. Working from that and working with any degree of doubt about whether the patient really has had as much immunization as he should have had, they are sprinkling the stuff over the community at a great rate. They are using 250 vials a month, I believe. I should not have thought there would have been much difference in the usage of anti-zoster-immunoglobulin from one place to another, unless perhaps our leukemia centers are more active and more aware of the availability of the product. Anti-rubella immunoglobulin hardly moves at all.

P.C. Das:

I would like to direct a question to Dr. Klein. You have visited Blood Banks in Holland, what do you think of continental standards? How do they perform?

R.E. Klein, Winston-Salem, NC, USA:

As I said, standards I talked about are those we use in the USA. I find that from country to country standards must differ. Allan Richardson Jones once said to me in his typical British accent: "Bob, when common sense interferes with the rules, to hell with the rules." When I inspected an US-army Blood Bank in the Panama Canal Zone, and they had no questions regarding malaria, they said: "Oh, but our donors have had malaria at least twice, all of them." So I said: "To hell with the rules." And we accredited them. Then I went to Alaska and a technician from a very small Indian village, isolated ten months out of the year, told me that hepatitis was endemic, that everybody had had it. What should she do if she cannot have donors with negative hepatitis? I said to myself (but not to her): "To hell with the rules." Your donor medical analysis being done in The Netherlands is unheard of, as far as I know. And yet it is an added dimension for donating a pint of blood. I cannot say that every nation should be following what we in the USA are doing. But on the other hand: If you want to, we would welcome the opportunity to come and visit you, send an inspector and see if you can attain accreditation as the Red Cross Blood Bank Groningen-Drenthe has.

W.L. Marsh:

Can I address a question to Dr. Klein about quality assurance of apparatus? Tell me, what data is there to show that there is a defect in the centrifuge, it does not run quite fast enough, that there is a slight fluctuation in the temperature of a waterbath, any data to show that that does indeed compromise the accuracy of the test we are doing?

R.E. Klein:

The truth of it is, many tests and many numerals that we recite in blood banking are – if you will excuse the expression – idiot rules. But you do have to have rules for the vast majority. You have recited for us a great many things that you do in your New York Blood Center. I would say those are fine for the New York Blood Center, but you would not apply those to a 50-bed hospital in Kentucky. It is in the small hospitals that you have to have rules. You have to say: "These numbers apply." If we get to your hospitals, the reagent quality control is different from what we would expect in a place such as Shifting Sands, Texas, Podunk, Wisconsin and so forth. We would not apply the same criteria at your huge Donor Center that we would at that small hospital.

W.L. Marsh:

That is of course a typical politician's reply. Is there any data to show that if my waterbath does not run at the correct temperature, this does compromise the tests I do? I am just curious. Is there any data to show that if you do Rheses-D typing at 32°C, you get a percentage of inaccuracies?

B.A. Myhre:

I am glad you brought that up, since it is a pet subject of mine. The question is: How do you get an accurate surface temperature? We went through some very interesting things with Rhesus slide boxes to find out that most surface-temperature thermometers are inaccurate. We did a very simple study: Varied the temperature through a large range, created our own dry box, and found that, using FDA standards, the anti-D serum would react with red cells in almost any suspension, from about 5% to about 50% – at which point you cannot see it, and would reproduce results at a range of 20°C to about 50°C. In that range, when you put the albumin on, it turns white and cooks. So, we came to the conclusion that anything beyond room temperature and below cooking of the albumin, and any red cell concentration that you can see, will give you an accurate response.

There were other things we got interested in: The dry bath. I must admit that I did bring this up as a possibility of measuring all the corners. One of my engineering friends said: "You must be out of your mind. Metal is metal, and metal transmits heat."

We checked and found a one degree difference all the way round. In waterbaths heated from below, water circulates. It would circle around and come back up, and therefore they are stirred. The temperature difference in the average waterbath, as long as you do not put a big flask or such in the middle of it, will be within one degree all the way around.

I have come to the conclusion that a lot of these things are a waste of time. We do them, although we should not waste our time doing it.

R.E. Klein:

We just went through a new Blood Center with all new centrifuges. Quite a lengthy procedure in trying to ascertain the best duration and revolution per minute, for a variety of component preparations. We found platelet production in particular was greatly influenced in varying ways of duration and speed. So I do think it is worthwhile to perform some quality control on equipment, as I have outlined. The same would be true for other pieces of equipment. I cannot agree that we should disregard the testing of each piece of equipment to assure that it is functioning as it is expected to function.

C.F. Högman, Uppsala, Sweden:

Could I raise the question of the impact of certain quality control? It makes a difference how frequent you select samples, for example, if you measure the pH of platelet concentrate, and do enough, you will find that some of them are below 6.0 after 72 hours and some are above. You may be satisfied if 75% of them are above 6.0, but you could use the information in a different way: You could say any platelet concentrate which is below 6.0 should be discarded and not used in the clinics. If you use it in that way, you have to test every sample that you are issuing, because you know for sure some of these untis will not meet the standards. I bring up this point, because I think this is quite an interesting and rather difficult situation we are in. I just took this as an example. If we look at the platelet concentrate, we could say that perhaps we should test every unit, for instance at 48 hours, and then discard those which do not meet a certain standard. In this way, we could improve quality. But this would mean we have to rely on a piece of tubing, because of course we cannot open the units.

C.Th. Smit Sibinga:

It is a very important issue and I fully agree with you. The point is that first you have to define your philosophy and then set your criteria. I have tried to give an outline based on what I have learned in recent years with respect to quality assurance. I went over the four premises set by WHO, which can be found in any GMP manual: safety, purity, potency and efficacy. In my presentation, I deliberately went no further than up to the element "potency", because "efficacy" is going to be dealt with tomorrow.

What one wants to know is, whatever product issued should really meet the standards of clinical efficacy. Therefore not only the standard in your Blood Bank weighs, but the clinical evaluation of the unit is of importance as well. In our region, as a standard for platelet concentrates, by agreement with the clinicians, one-hour increments are monitored. That gives us a feedback on how things fit into the criteria you referred to regarding pH and platelet functions. It is not purely the word criterion and the cut-off level of 6.0; we should refine and precisely define these things.

B.A. Myhre:

What you bring up is an extremely interesting point. Again, it would be very nice if one could analyze, just prior to transfusion, every component. But we cannot because of the volume, and because of the break in the sterility.

In my misspent middle age I have fallen under the sway of a number of quality control engineers, who, now I find, are being called system analysts and system operation technologists. They worked out some fascinating formulae, based on previous records of how many units had been known to fail. From this one can work out statistically how many should be checked to make certain to pick up one that will fail. Basically, what it translates into is the more failures you are seeing, the more often you ought to check. The less failures you see, the less often you ought to check. This ties in with what I was saying to Dr. Klein. No, I do not feel we should stop checking equipment. However, if we have something like a dry bath, where the heat transmission cannot vary, unless the basic laws of physics are violated, we should not bother checking that. On the other hand, when we have a thermostat that is controlling the heat of this dry bath, that can fail easily, we need to check much more often.

Ch.A. Schiffer, Baltimore, USA:

I enjoyed your comments very much. It is really quite true that the failure rate in terms of pH of platelet concentrates can vary by a significant figure. It is a lot lower than 25% in good Blood Banks. At 72 hours it is probably a lot higher in poor Blood Banks, which do not pay very much attention to platelet concentrate preparation. It is a very reasonable suggestion to test pH prior to transfusion, although I think we might be the only place I know of, that actually does that with platelets that are 72 hours old. I also know of no Blood Bank to drop their price by 25%, if they find that 25% of their 72-hour platelets are in fact totally non-viable.

In fact, they probably make a lot more money because the patient has to be re-transfused. This is not being facetious, that happens very commonly. With respect to bacterial contamination of platelet concentrate, this is extraordinarily rare. I come from the institution that became famous for describing that phenomenon. We stopped culturing our platelets years ago. Frankly, clinically it is an incredibly rare phenomenon, if it happes at all anymore.

C.Th. Smit Sibinga:

If you go over the figures which Dr. Das has presented, you may have noticed that there were none positive for platelets so far. That points to the fact that we do not find anything. Still, we are doing it. We have to reconsider where to go from here, or alternatively raise the question: How much is enough? Where does overdoing things start?

C.F. Högman:

Just one last comment. I think in many respects our quality assurance, our quality control is rather arbitrary. This reminds me of a story. It is late in the night, and there is a man coming down the street. He spots a man under a street lamp, looking for something and asks: "What are you looking for?" "I am looking for my door key", says the man. The first man starts to help in the search for the door key. "Was it really here that you lost your key?" he asks. "Oh no, it was over there, but it is to dark over there", the man replied. I think that quite often in science, we find parallels to this story.

III. Personnel

JOB DESCRIPTIONS, COMPETENCY TESTING AND SELECTION OF PERSONNEL

H. v.d. Meulen

INTRODUCTION

Taking into account the limitations with which I feel myself confronted, my objective is to stimulate thinking about a field with which one might be less familiar than the medical or technological one. First a few remarks will be made about the field of human resource management in general, followed by some statements concerning manpower planning, what job descriptions are and what purposes they may serve, and some statements about personnel selection.

HUMAN RESOURCE MANAGEMENT

The topics mentioned in this contribution, manpower planning, job description and selection of personnel are belonging to the field described in handbooks as personnel management or human resources management. Human resources management can be defined as the planning, attraction, selection, retention, development, utilization and dismissal of human resources in order to achieve individual as well as organizational objectives. From the definition we learn in the first place that human resources management does not concern exclusively the objectives of the organization or the objectives of the individual, but on the whole will have to find a balance between the two. Easy when the objectives are the same: a little difficult when the objectives donot coincide for 100%; very difficult when they seem to be opposed to each other.

In the second place the definition tells us that human resources management containes a number of activities from attraction to dismissal, which influence each other like other activities in the organization. Each of these activities can reinforce the result of the previous one or annihilate that result. Imagine that after planning how much blood will be needed, calling up the right number of donors, taking the blood with all the necessary precautions, the further processing of the blood is done in such a negligent way that its quality is lost. What a waste and what a loss of energy! Yet one sometimes gets the impression when, after a careful job description, planning, recruiting and selection process the newly appointed employee in the organization (our organization?) goes to waste because of a lack of adequate introduction, training, supervising or other elements of the human resource management process, the organization values its human resources less than bloodbanks value their blood.

Working conditions, for example, under which human beings fulfill their jobs at any level of the organization, future skills and knowledge organizations expect from their present and prospective employees, are often poorly defined. Whenever the results of a manpower planning process shows descrepancies between those expectations, the organization should take adequate measures which might, for example, include training, personnel development programs, activities concerned with restructuring the contents of jobs or improving working conditions.

JOB DESCRIPTIONS

Before any manpower or human resource planning can be carried out, management should first define what work is to be performed and how the many tasks can be divided and allocated into manageable work units, which we call jobs. Such an assignment of tasks to jobs in commonly known as a "job design" reflected in a job description. A job description is a written statement of what the jobholder does, how the job is done and why it is done, telling us what the tasks are which have to be performed. How this relates to the behaviour necessary to perform the job in the right way. Why is the job relating to other jobs and the overall organizational goal(s). The information which the job description provides can be used to determine what knowledge, skills, abilities and other specifications are required to perform the job. These so called job specifications can be of great help in recruiting, selection, introduction, training and supervising activities. From the various techniques available to obtain information about different jobs the ones which are most used will be mentioned.

1. Direct observation

The analist actually observes the individual performing the job and records observations while doing so. This method is very suitable for jobs that require a great deal of manual, standardised, short cycle activities which occur at regular intervals. It is less appropriate if not impossible for jobs, in which some elements of the complete job cycle occur at infrequent and perhaps unpredictable intervals and for jobs that require a great deal of mental activity and concentration.

2. The interview

The interview is probably the most commonly used technique for establishing the tasks, duties and behaviour necessary for both standardised or non-standardised activities and for physical as well as mental work. Because the job holder acts as his or her own observer in the interview, he or she can report activities and behaviours that will not often be observed, as well as activities that occur over a long time span. The success of this technique is partly dependent on the skill of the interviewer. Training of the analist in interviewing techniques as well as thorough advance planning should precede the actual interview. For reasons of reliability and efficiency, the interviewer should follow a protocolled interview that systematically covers the information to be gathered during the interview. A danger may be that the job holder consciously or unconsciously exaggerates the importance of the job. This danger, however, can be overcome by interviewing more than one of the same job holders and also one or more of their direct supervisors. A disadvantage is that this method is very time consuming.

3. Using a questionnaire or checklist

Questionnaires are usually standardised and provide either checking items that apply to a job, or rating items in terms of their relevance to the job in question. This method is most likely the least costly for collecting job analysis data. Where there are many workers in a job, questionnaires provide a wide coverage, that would be very expensive and time consuming to obtain by any other method. It requires, however, a well designed questionnaire or checklist and even then there is a danger that a respondee will either not complete it, complete it inaccurately or take an excessively long time to return it.

4. Job performance

This method is only appropriate for jobs that the analist can readily learn.

General opinion of specialists in this field nowadays is that probably the most effective way of obtaining job analysis data is the combination of direct observation and interview.

The information, concerning a job which is obtained by one or more of the above mentioned methods, has to be sorted out and converted into an effective job description. An effective job description should enable anybody who does not know the job by own experience, to form an idea of the job and its requirements. Along with the data for job descriptions the job analysis should generate job specifications, which represent a statement of the human qualifications required to perform the job. Among the qualifications that may be specified are:

1. educational standards;
2. experience required;
3. skills required;
4. physical requirements;
5. certifications or licenses required.

It is sometimes believed that jobs are static entities. We should, however, recognize that most jobs are more dynamic than their descriptions from two points of view:

1. activities in most organizations will gradually change, owing to technical changes or other reasons;
2. regardless of the description of the job, the human being performing it will moderate the contents of the job.

Regularly updating of the information necessary to make a job description and concerning the contents of a job may serve a number of purposes:

1. Tasks comprising a job will change from time to time due to technological or other reasons. Up to date job analysis may provide the organization with an indication if and when a job needs re-designing because of task content changes. For example, technological changes may reduce considerably the time required to perform certain tasks in donor centre, laboratory or component division and make it necessary to give the job holder other duties or additional training for new tasks to keep him or her busy doing a full-time job.

2. Identifying the work to be performed in each job provides an extremely important basis for planning the organization's human resources.

3. Describing accurately what each job comprises is essential for recruiting and selection.

4. Job analysis provides valuable data for performance appraisal, since it helps to permit a comparison between an individual's job performance and the tasks required to be carried out as specified in the job design.

5. Job analysis provides a basis for training and development. In order to train an individual we first need a definition of the tasks he is expected to carry out and if possible a description of the way in which they should be carried out.

6. Job analysis data are often used in relation to salary and wage systems. Basic for evaluating and comparing jobs for wage and salary purposes is a clear statement of what each job entails.

The Dutch Ministry of Social Affairs has recently published a survey concerning the use and adaptation of job analysis systems in organizations in 1980. From this we learn that in only 23% of the labour organizations a job analysis system is used, mostly in relation to remuneration systems. In only 25% of the organizations which use a job analysis system, thus in only 6% of the total labour organizations in the Netherlands, a job analysis system is used for other purposes. This so called multicharacter concerns selection, training and personnel development activities.

Our conclusion might be at this point that job analysis up to now is regarded for too little as a tool of management.

PERSONNEL SELECTION

Organizations use a wide array of selecting decisions regarding applicants from outside the organization. Tests, biographical data and interview represent these major categories. There is considerable diversity of specific techniques within each category, generally referred to as predictors. A predictor is valid when the information it provides about applicants is related to their future successful performance of the job. Even the most sophisticated psychological tests cannot be a perfect predictor as it cannot include circumstantial factors of the job, style of supervision, reactions of collegues and many other variables. For less sophisticated techniques this is even more true. Despite the fact that the selection interviews probably contribute little validity to the selection decision, it continues to be used. It is clear that no amount of additional evidence of the lack of validity will alter the role of the interview in selection. Future research should obviously be directed at understanding the mechanism of the interview and improving interview technology. The results of recent research indicate that only structured interviews generate information that different people interviewing the same interviewee can agree about. Will interviewers be able to make predictions about the future job behaviour of the interviewee than they should be able to evaluate information obtained from the interviewee in terms of what the interviewee will be able to do in the job in question.

The view that the selection process should no longer be looked upon as a oneside activity from the organization towards the applicant but a matching process between applicant and job, calls for another attitude of the interviewer. The hiring decision in this view is not the end but the beginning of a process in which employees and organization systematically keep up a continuous discussion which has as its ultimate goal a job performance of the qualitative standard our organization demands.

TRAINING PROGRAMS FOR BLOOD BANK PERSONNEL

B.A. Myhre

The blood bank faces a serious problem when dealing with the training of new personnel. These personnel are to be performing in an area in which no errors are allowable, at least as far as the final product is concerned. This requires a type of training and also mental discipline that is not usually included in many of the training courses. Further, the blood bank personnel must function as a team. It is not possible for only one of them to operate a complex machine and turn out results as needed. The team is all involved in drawing donors, typing blood, preparing components, and in performing cross matches. Errors, or a poor work response in any one section can reflect on the whole organization, and can conceivably endanger a patient's life. Therefore all persons must perform their own jobs perfectly, and must also know the problems of the other areas so that they may work together as a well functioning whole. All of these interactions require knowledge of the other areas of the laboratory, and a very detailed knowledge of one's own particular area. This can be obtained only through extra training. It is absolutely necessary that a blood bank provides this training for all levels of individuals involved with blood. It would seem that this training could be done adequately in formal university programs. In many cases it is, but the blood bank offers a unique amalgamation of available material, interested instructors, and a feeling of enthusiasm which can be lacking in some of the other programs. Further, many newly hired employees, have not obtained this higher level of specialized knowledge in their previous places of employment or training, and therefore must be trained not only in the rudements of blood banking, but how those methods are applied in a particular institution. Further from a legal standpoint, a unified and documented initial training program assures the courts that all employees were following the same technics at any particular time. To provide a baseline of knowledge required for all employees, an initial in-house training program is essential.

For this program to work, however, one must define the target population which will be trained, the training goals, and the method that will be used to evaluate their training. To illustrate these points, I have outlined the goals for an in-house course of instruction, as I see them, for all levels of persons to be trained. This includes new employees who have just been hired by a free-standing blood center, or students possibly on loan from some other institution for specialized training. The goals are broad generalities which state what the purposes of the learning experience are. From this set of goals, a series of objectives can be written that are clearly stated subunits of each of the goals, and which must be directly quantifiable in some manner. A well written objective almost always leads directly to the question to test if it has been achieved.

Before we can begin to state goals, it is necessary to break down the target population of learners into sub-populations. The classification I propose is as follows:

1. Donor Recruiter – a person responsible for contacting and scheduling donors desiring to give blood.
2. Phlebotomy Nurse – the nurse performing the phlebotomies.
3. Supervisory Nurse – a nurse supervising the phlebotomists.
4. Student technologist – a student studying general laboratory technology.
5. Student Blood Bank Technologist – a student specializing in blood banking; may already be graduate technologist.
6. Working Technologist – a technologist who is trained and performing routine work in the blood bank.
7. Supervisory Technologist – a technologist who is responsible for supervising other technologists in a section, or who has special knowledge, i.e. runs a consultation service.
8. Administrative Technologists – a technologist who is responsible for the general administrative operation of the laboratory.
9. Practicing physician – a clinician interested in the use of blood for transfusing patients.
10. Laboratory physician – a general laboratory physician responsible for a blood transfusion service.
11. Medical Director – a director of the blood bank responsible for donor bleeding, processing, and other medical functions.

Of course not all of these positions will be in any one blood bank. Some of the positions may not be used, or some of them may be combined; but for purposes of discussion, they will be presented in this form.

After the target populations have been defined, the various goals of training can be written. Most of these goals will be the same for all employees, however, each sub-population needs to achieve these goals in varying degrees. Therefore it is necessary to define how much knowledge of any particular goal is needed by each category of employee. Fortunately, this quantitation has already been done for us. A study of the Cognitive Domaine culminated in a book which lists the criteria, and gives their definitions. In Bloom's "Taxonomy of Educational Objectives" (2) these categories are listed in part as follows:

1.00 Knowledge - recall of specifics, universals, methods, processes, patterns, structure, or setting.

1.11 - knowledge of terminology alone.

1.12 - knowledge of specific facts.
1.21 - knowledge of conventions.
1.23 - knowledge of classification and categories.
1.31 - knowledge of principles and generalizations.
2.00 Comprehension - know what is being communicated and make use of the material.
3.00 Application - use of abstractions in particular and concrete situations.
4.00 Analysis - breakdown of a communication into its constituent elements or parts such that the relative hierarchy of ideas is made clear.
5.00 Synthesis - putting together of elements and parts so as to form a whole.
6.00 Evaluation - judgements about the value of material and methods for given purposes.

From these goals, training categories, and taxonomic values we may construct a twodimensional matrix of the desired educational goals. This matrix is shown in Figure 1. The desired goals are listed as rows on the y axis. The columns on the x axis show the employee positions which need training. The rest of the chart is filled with the individual taxonomic classifications of each goal as it applies to each job. As has been previously stated, it is my feeling that a certain exposure to all these goals is needed for all the jobs, however, the amount of knowledge required will vary. For example, a donor recruiter should know a considerable amount about donor scheduling methods, (level = 5.0) while the laboratory technologist needs only to know that there can be a problem (1.23). On the other hand, a recruiter needs only to know that an antiglobulin test exists and is used in cross matching (1.11); while the technologist needs to know most of the variables pertaining to this reaction (5.0).

Once the goals required for each job have been defined, and the taxonomic classifications have been developed, a series of detailed training objectives must be developed. Each of these objectives should be small and clearly stated. A number of objectives will be needed to clearly define one goal. The objectives must be properly defined in a quantitative manner. For example, it is not enough to use as an objective the statement "the student will have an appreciation of the accuracy required to do a cross match". This is a goal. Rather, the objective must be defined as "the student will demonstrate the accuracy required for a cross match by performing 10 cross matches while being observed and making no errors in sample identification, tube labelling, specimen transfer, reagent addition or final reading of the reaction".

After the objectives have been written, it is necessary only to decide the best way to teach these skills. Here one should be guided by the principle that <u>a person does not teach, a student learns</u>. Therefore any method is acceptable as long as the student learns. Some skills, especially motor ones such as performing cross matches, venepunctures, making components, etc. can be taught by supervised laboratory work, continuous loop films,

Fig. 1

SERVICE	Recruiter	Phlebotomy Nurse	Supervisory Nurse	Med. Tech. Student	SBB Student	Working Med. Tech.	Supervising Med. Tech.	Admin. Med. Tech.	Practicing Physician	Lab Physician	B.B. Med. Director
RECRUITING											
1. Basic strategies in donor recruitment	5.0	1.11	3.0	1.11	1.31	1.23	2.0	3.0	1.21	2.0	4.0
2. Appropriate scheduling of mobile collection units	4.0	1.11	3.0	1.11	1.31	1.23	2.0	3.0	1.21	2.0	4.0
3. Principles of motivating donors	6.0	2.0	3.0	1.11	1.31	1.23	2.0	3.0	2.0	2.0	5.0
4. Accounting methods used for blood donation	3.0	1.11	2.0	1.11	1.31	1.23	1.23	2.0	1.11	2.0	3.0
DONOR BLEEDING											
1. Standards of donation	2.0	4.0	5.0	1.21	1.31	1.31	2.0	3.0	1.21	3.0	5.0
2. Acceptance and Rejection criteria	3.0	4.0	5.0	1.21	1.31	1.31	2.0	3.0	1.21	3.0	5.0
3. Counseling of donors as to abnormalities	3.0	4.0	5.0	1.21	1.31	1.31	2.0	3.0	1.31	4.0	5.0
4. Correct venepuncture technic	1.0	4.0	5.0	1.23	1.23	1.23	1.23	1.23	1.23	2.0	2.0
5. Donor reactions - Diagnosis - Types	1.23	3.0	4.0	1.21	1.23	1.23	1.23	1.23	1.23	2.0	4.0
6. Donor reactions - Treatment	1.23	4.0	5.0	1.23	1.23	1.23	1.23	1.23	1.23	3.0	5.0
7. Apheresis technics	2.0	4.0	5.0	1.23	2.0	1.23	2.0	3.0	1.23	3.0	5.0
8. Anticoagulant solutions and containers	1.23	2.0	3.0	1.23	3.0	2.0	3.0	4.0	1.23	3.0	5.0
IMMUNOGENETICS											
1. Basic immunology knowledge	1.11	1.11	1.11	1.23	3.0	3.0	4.0	5.0	1.23	4.0	6.0
antigens, antibodies, & complement	1.11	1.11	1.11	1.31	4.0	4.0	6.0	5.0	1.23	4.0	6.0
2. Tissue compatibility	1.11	1.11	1.11	1.31	4.0	4.0	5.0	5.0	3.0	4.0	6.0
3. Basic genetics	1.11	1.11	1.11	2.0	4.0	3.0	5.0	5.0	3.0	4.0	6.0
4. Red cell, platelet, and leukocyte groups	1.11	1.11	1.11	2.0	4.0	3.0	4.0	5.0	2.0	4.0	5.0
5. Basic serologic technics	1.11	1.11	1.11	1.21	2.0	3.0	5.0	4.0	2.0	3.0	5.0
6. Hepatitis and S.T.S. testing	2.0	1.23	3.0	1.21	2.0	3.0	3.0	4.0	2.0	3.0	5.0
7. Automated technics	1.11	1.11	1.21	1.23	3.0	3.0	3.0	5.0	1.21	3.0	5.0
COMPONENT PREPARATION											
1. Type components	2.0	2.0	2.0	1.21	2.0	3.0	3.0	4.0	2.0	3.0	4.0
2. Methods of preparation	1.11	1.11	2.0	2.0	3.0	4.0	4.0	5.0	1.23	3.0	5.0
STORAGE AND TRANSPORTATION											
1. Current methods of storage for most components	1.23	1.21	1.23	2.0	2.0	3.0	4.0	5.0	1.23	3.0	5.0
Frozen blood	1.23	1.21	1.23	2.0	2.0	3.0	4.0	5.0	1.23	3.0	5.0
2. Methods of inventory control	2.0	1.21	1.21	2.0	3.0	3.0	3.0	5.0	1.21	3.0	5.0

COMPATIBILITY TESTING											
1. Patient specimens	1.0	1.11	1.11	2.0	4.0	4.0	4.0	4.0	3.0	4.0	5.0
2. Principles and procedures for most common technics	1.0	1.11	1.11	2.0	4.0	4.0	5.0	5.0	2.0	4.0	5.0
The antiglobulin test	1.11	1.11	1.11	2.0	4.0	4.0	5.0	5.0	2.0	4.0	5.0
Abbreviated vs. true crossmatches	1.21	1.11	1.11	2.0	4.0	4.0	5.0	5.0	2.0	4.0	5.0
Enzymes and Lectins	1.11	1.11	1.11	2.0	4.0	4.0	5.0	5.0	1.21	4.0	5.0
PROBLEM STUDIES											
1. Principles of solving problem crossmatches	1.11	1.11	1.11	2.0	4.0	4.0	4.0	5.0	1.23	3.0	5.0
2. Use of Rare Donor files	2.0	1.23	1.31	2.0	4.0	4.0	5.0	4.0	1.23	3.0	4.0
3. Transfusion reactions - diagnosis & types	1.11	1.21	1.21	1.23	3.0	3.0	5.0	4.0	3.0	4.0	5.0
4. Transfusion reactions - Treatment	1.11	1.21	1.23	1.23	3.0	3.0	4.0	4.0	3.0	4.0	5.0
ADMINISTRATION AND PRODUCTION MANAGEMENT											
1. Quality Control Programs	1.0	1.11	1.21	1.21	3.0	2.0	3.0	5.0	1.21	3.0	5.0
2. Time and Motion Technics	1.0	1.21	2.0	1.21	2.0	3.0	3.0	5.0	1.11	2.0	4.0
3. Instrumentation	1.1	1.11	1.11	1.21	2.0	3.0	3.0	5.0	1.11	3.0	4.0
4. Personnel Policies & Job descriptions	1.21	1.11	4.0	1.21	2.0	3.0	3.0	4.0	1.21	4.0	4.0
5. Records	2.0	1.23	2.0	4.0	5.0	5.0	5.0	6.0	2.0	5.0	6.0
6. Labelling	1.31	2.0	3.0	4.0	5.0	5.0	5.0	6.0	2.0	5.0	6.0
CONSULTATION											
Use of correct blood components in following situations											
1. Blood transfusion ordering and practices	2.0	1.31	2.0	2.0	4.0	4.0	4.0	4.0	3.0	4.0	4.0
2. Coagulation disorder	1.31	1.31	2.0	2.0	3.0	3.0	4.0	4.0	3.0	4.0	5.0
3. HDN	1.31	1.31	2.0	2.0	3.0	3.0	4.0	4.0	3.0	4.0	5.0
4. Neonatal transfusions	1.21	1.31	2.0	2.0	3.0	3.0	4.0	4.0	3.0	4.0	5.0
5. Massive Trauma	1.21	1.31	2.0	2.0	3.0	3.0	4.0	4.0	3.0	4.0	5.0
6. Auto Immune Hemolytic Anemia	1.21	1.31	2.0	2.0	3.0	3.0	4.0	4.0	3.0	5.0	6.0
7. The Problem patient	1.21	1.31	2.0	2.0	3.0	3.0	4.0	4.0	3.0	5.0	6.0
8. Follow up of transfusion reactions	1.21	1.31	2.0	2.0	3.0	3.0	4.0	4.0	3.0	5.0	6.0
EDUCATION											
1. In-service training	4.0	3.0	4.0	2.0	4.0	4.0	5.0	5.0	4.0	6.0	6.0
2. Continuing education for hospital staff physicians	3.0	2.0	2.0	2.0	3.0	3.0	4.0	3.0	4.0	6.0	6.0
3. Methods of Inspection and Accreditation	3.0	2.0	4.0	2.0	3.0	3.0	5.0	6.0	3.0	5.0	5.0
RESEARCH											
Personally motivated and determined	4.0	2.0	4.0	2.0	4.0	3.0	5.0	4.0	2.0	4.0	6.0

computer assisted education, video tape and movies. Recruiting skills may require lectures, on-the-job training, role model playing, supervision and coaching, and discussion groups. Almost all skills will require some lecture and reading assignments. However, one should always remember the technics of teaching are less important than the definition of what is to be taught. One should never be caught in the trap of teaching methodologies. There is always more than one way to teach anything, and it depends more on the student than on the subject manner as to which method is best. A teacher should be enough of a Machiavellian scholar to use the best method for that student at that particular time. Certainly, some of the training will not be formal. Much of it will be on-the-job or will be by experience, but nevertheless, the listing of goals will at least show what is needed for the full training of the particular individual, and will demonstrate when the training goals have been achieved.

A final type of teaching is used relatively infrequently, but is especially powerful. This is the method of Socratic discussions. In this method, the student is asked questions, and the answers are then guided by further questions and discussion. This method allows the student to develop his own base of knowledge founded on already present knowledge which the instructor has caused the student to re-evaluate, and to reform into a new series of working concepts. This type of teaching often produces knowledge with the longest recall period.

At the end of the learning period, an examination of some kind must be given to document that the student has really learned all these skills. This is needed to satisfy university regulations, state licensing standards, and legal requirements. If the objectives have been defined clearly and precisely; the extent and type of testing usually is self evident. It is only necessary then to write the questions, and to administer the examination.

It is best to use a comprehensive examination which has been tested repeatedly on a large group of people. This of course means that a copy of the examination probably is available in the students "scribs" and is used for study. There is nothing wrong with this. If the examination tests for the basic goals, then there is no reason why the students shouldnot study from an old copy of the examination. If they are able to learn and understand the questions, and prove this knowledge by answering the questions correctly, then they have achieved the objectives of learning. The purpose of the examination is to prove that the goals and objectives have been achieved; not to serve as a platform for failure. If an employee fails, then the instruction should be repeated and the examination readministered. If there is a subsequent failure, then the employee should be questioned as to why the failure occurred. The employee should be considered unsatisfactory only after several failures with no subsequent improvement.

After the examination has been taken, the final score should be retained in the blood banks files. It may be necessary at a later date to certify to one of the licensing or certifying groups that the instruction was taken. It is embarassing to do this if one does not even remember the employees name much less the performance on the examination. Therefore, the records should be retained.

REFERENCES

1. Bailey, A.A. Education in the New Age, Lucis Pub. Co., N.Y. 1971.
2. Bloom. Taxonomy of Educational Objectives". David McKay & Co., Inc. N.Y., 1956.
3. Downie, N.M.. Fundamentals of Measurement: Techniques and Practices, Oxford Univ. Press, N.Y. 1958.
4. Highet, G.. The Art of Teaching, Vintage Books, N.Y. 1957.
5. Popham, W.J., Baker, E.L. Establishing Instructional Goals, Prentice-Hall Inc., Englewood Cliffs, N.J. 1970
6. Popham, W.J., Baker, E.L. Planning an Instructional Sequence, Prentice-Hall Inc., Englewood Cliffs, N.J. 1970.
7. Tyler, R.W. Basic Principles of Curriculum and Instruction, Univ. of Chi. Press, Chicago 1949.

CONTINUOUS EDUCATION IN BLOOD BANKING AND BLOOD TRANSFUSION PRACTICE

S.R. Hollán

Continuous education of the staff of bloodtransfusion services (BTS) and hospital blood banks, as well as postgraduate teaching of physicians and surgeons in bloodtransfusion practice represents major tasks of bloodtransfusion services throughout the world. The sharp increase in basic scientific information on structure and function of blood cells and plasma constituents, the newly developed methods in processing of blood components and plasma fractionation, the advances in immunology, blood group serology, coagulation and cryobiology, the ever changing aspects of the clinical application of blood transfusion necessitate a regular house-staff and professional staff education program even in the most advanced bloodtransfusion centres. This is also of paramount importance in developing countries where the shortage of trained personnel represents the main limiting factor in the development of their national bloodtransfusion services.

It is a most surprising fact that even in countries with a highly developed health service there is no adequate systematic training in the theoretical basis and clinical application of bloodtransfusion for medical students and residents. A number of the senior staff in some departments of surgery, obstetrics, gynaecology, medicine and paediatrics is still obsessed by the myths of whole bloodtransfusion and some other now outdated concepts. Regular postgraduate education of medical residents and senior staff of all medical institutions is needed to achieve a scientifically better based, safer, more rational, and cost-effective use of blood.

The optimal basic training for the director of a bloodtransfusion centre is still a debated problem in many parts of the world. I hold the opinion that the director should be preferably a physician, trained in the laboratory and clinical aspects of haematology, immunology and bloodtransfusion. Advances in these fields of biomedicine have progressed so rapidly that most physicians and surgeons find it difficult to keep up with the changes in the basic concepts which underline the everyday practice of bloodtransfusion. However, they will only consult the blood bank physician if he is known to have a good scientific reputation and to be well skilled in both laboratory and clinical problems of haemotherapy. This is also a prerequisite of setting up adequate postgraduate teaching programs in bloodtransfusion.

The aims, trends and scopes of the training programs of the professional and house staff have to be adapted 1) to the peculiar aspects of transfusion therapy: to the interaction between the donor and the recipient, and 2) to the basic functions of the bloodtransfusion service. This latter comprises:

- collection, separation, processing and distribution of blood and its derivatives;
- application of laboratory tests;
- advice on clinical usage;
- training and teaching, and
- research and development.

The first three tasks are universally accepted but the two latter ones have not been included into the basic tasks of many centres. In contrast, in my opinion training and teaching, as well as an active research program are essential features of an efficient bloodtransfusion service. The best way of keeping pace with and having a good command of our current understanding of the biological basis of haemotherapy and the most recent advances in both technology and clinical practice is to teach. The blood centre staff has to participate actively in disseminating information in this increasingly important and rapidly advancing field of medicine. Fundamental research is to contribute information to the fields of science related to blood and is a sine qua non for the development of new techniques in processing blood and blood derivatives and for the scientific evaluation of the results of routine tests.

The first basic tasks of a BTS is aimed at producing adequate amounts of safe and effective blood components and plasma products. A regional centre has to provide whole blood, blood components and plasma fractions of guaranteed biological activity for the whole area to be supplied. The staff has to be aware of the fact that the quality of the final product depends upon the quality of their performance in donor selection, collection of blood or plasma, and the handling of the source material throughout processing. As a consequence, the production, diagnostic and safety aspects of a bloodtransfusion centre are not separated but integrated elements.

In setting up a National Blood Program calculations have to be made of the amount of blood and blood derivatives needed. The optimum size of a donor panel comprises seven donors per one emergency bed and the recruitment of around 2 to 5% of the total population as regular donors. In Hungary 5.8% of the population is regular voluntary donor. It is also indispensable to have a panel of donors with rare blood groups and a panel of donors with high levels of specific antibodies. When planning the size of the blood donor panel the need for different components has to be approximated.

In planning the size of the plasmapheresis and cell-apheresis panels, the need for plasma for specific plasma proteins and for platelet concentrates has to be calculated. Granulocyte donors are recruited most frequently from family members of the recipient. The final size of the specific donor panels has to be continuously re-evaluated and revised according to the actual judgement of the real needs.

In many countries, especially in the developing countries, there is a deficiency in whole blood and blood derivatives. But even in countries with highly developed bloodtransfusion services, the amount of blood and plasma collected, has to be increased year by year. New methods have arisen which consume blood voraciously. Let me list some of these fairly new fields of indication. Coronary bypass surgery alone may raise by 26% the need for whole blood. Emergency direct coronary arterial revascularization, infarctectomy, aneurysmectomy, repair of ruptured ventricular septum, liver surgery, surgery of cerebral ischaemia, as well as major surgery in traumatology and orthopaedics, like hemipelvectomy and implantation of joint prostheses, all consume substantial amounts of blood. Extremely high amounts of platelets are needed for patients on prolonged extracorporeal oxygenation by a membrane oxygenator and for patients on "artificial liver". Great amounts of platelets and sometimes granulocytes are needed for patients on aggressive chemotherapy and after bone marrow transplantation.

When new operative procedures, like coronary bypass surgery are being initiated in a region, a thorough consideration has to be given to immediate and projected blood requirements. The same is true for all other newly arising fields of indication. The bloodtransfusion centre will only be able to meet the quantitatively and qualitatively increasing demands if the director or an expert of the staff will fully understand the basic principles and the hazards involved in the newly applied diagnostic or therapeutic procedures. And that is why continuous postgraduate training is indispensable.

There are three ways of providing more blood products:

- to bleed more donors;
- to have a more widespread use of plasmapheresis and cell-apheresis; and, last but not least
- to achieve optimal use of the collected fresh blood by component production.

The increase of the number of all voluntary, unpaid blood donation necessitates much work including propaganda, organization and recruitment. Consequently a training program has to include principles and practice of donor propaganda and recruitment as well as motivation of blood donation. You can never give a magic guideline in this subject, you have to find the best argument which will differ from time to time, and from place to place. Attracting new donors, especially unpaid voluntary donors accepting to undergo plasma and/or cell-apheresis requires broad educational efforts. While explaining the details of new needs in modern haemotherapy to the public of potential donors, it has to be stressed continuously that for those who need it, blood derivatives are as important as water supply for the community. Blood donors represent a natural focus for continuing education and dissemination of information, since they have already elected to join the donor ranks.

A training program of the staff of bloodtransfusion centres has to include also new methods of improving the organization of donor sessions, the preparation and use of mobile equipment and the application of new technologies to decrease the number and increase the efficiency of performances of staff participating at a session. Detailed instructions should repeatedly be given on incidents and accidents, hazards and contra-indications of blood donation. Thorough practical training has to be given on new improved techniques of collection of specific components as well as in techniques of giving bloodtransfusions. The participants in postgraduate training have to learn the theoretical basis and the practice of new techniques in blood and plama donation, cell separation, preservation and plasma fractionation. Basic biological and biophysical considerations and methodology of preservation of blood cells in the liquid and frozen state should be dealt with in details.

The staff has to be trained not only to use the most recent methods of plasmapheresis and cell-apheresis for obtaining high amounts of plasma or cell concentrates from donors, but in addition, they have to be acquainted with the therapeutic use of intensive plasma- and cell-apheresis.

Much has to be learned about new aspects of risks of transferring diseases by blood and derivatives, and about the preventive measures to avoid these hazards.

Due time should be spent to teach preparation and maintenance of equipment, devices and instruments associated with collection, processing, storage and administration of bloodtransfusion. Detailed instructions have to be given on minimum requirements for equipment, reagents, anticoagulants, sterilization procedures, and for the control tests evaluating the quality, biological activity and viability of the final products. A basic principle to be respected throughout the training is that one should never compromise between quality and quantity. The effectiveness of the education program is being controlled by frequent monitoring of the preparations produced by the trainees and by proficiency tests of their laboratory work.

Lectures shall be given on new aspects of structure, function, kinetics and viability of blood cells, which in fact define their optimum storage conditions. Participants have to learn to estimate cell survival. They have to be acquainted with the structure, function and the fractionation of plasma proteins.

Blood group serology represents of course the most important subject of the training. ABO, Lewis, Ii, Rh system and other RBC antigens have to be learned in theory and practice, as well as RBC allo- and autoantibodies and red cell incompatibility in vitro and in vivo. All participants of the course have to be acquainted with the platelet, lymphocyte, granulocyte, endothelial cell, macrophage and serum protein antigens and their respective antibodies as well as with the complement system. They have to learn how to prepare test sera, Coombs sera and cell panels for blood group serology. Blood groups and problems of parentage and identity are being reviewed briefly. Practical training enables the trainees to achieve good command of the application and evaluation of laboratory tests and gain some knowledge on the principles of automation.

Quality control represents another core subject of the training course.

We also find it important to teach the theory and practice of epidemiology and the prevention of transmittable diseases, as well as the epidemiology of non-infectious diseases prevailing in the area to be supplied with blood and derivatives.

Lectures on recent concepts of haemostasis and practical training of the methods applied in diagnostics and treatment of haemorragic diseases and thrombosis are to be included in the training program. Possibility shall be given during the training course to become acquainted with the methods of the production and use of plasma fractions with haemostatic activity.

Detailed lectures are to be given on indications of bloodtransfusion with special attention to component therapy, use and misuse of blood. Theoretical basis and practical aspects of the treatment of hypovolaemic shock and hazards of massive transfusion shall be discussed. Quantity and quality of blood components needed for extracorporeal circulation and haemodialysis shall also be included. To achieve optimum use of blood, detailed information has to be given on the use of plasma expanders and electrolyte solutions, and different plasma proteins, as well as a concise overview on artificial oxygen-carrying systems.

Blood centres often have to face the difficulties in finding compatible blood for patients with autoimmune diseases and this is why it is important to become acquainted with the pathophysiology, diagnostics and treatment of autoimmune diseases with special emphasis on haemotherapy and intensive plasmapheresis applied with success in the treatment of this heterogeneous group of diseases.

Neonates and infants are not small adults. Consequently, the program has to include the special aspects of haemotherapy in infancy and childhood: the pathophysiology, diagnostics, treatment and prevention of haemolytic diseases of the newborn, the technique of exchange transfusion and the treatment of the haemorrhagic disease of the newborn, and substitution therapy in immune deficiency.

Everybody involved in the production of blood and blood derivates, as well as those involved in the application of haemotherapy has to be fully aware of all hazards and complications of bloodtransfusion, the diagnosis, treatment, laboratory investigation, the prevention and also the legal aspects involved in bloodtransfusion.

Last but not least, management, financing, cost/benefit ratios and developmental work in the BTS shall be an integral part of the training program.

I have summarized the most important subjects of a postgraduate training, as taught at our postgraduate courses, including the six months' training course organized by WHO in our National Institute of Haematology and Blood Transfusion for experts in bloodtransfusion from fifteen developing countries. It gave us real satisfaction to hear that most of our students became heads of bloodtransfusion centres in their homeland.

The organization of postgraduate education is based on the principles of organization of our service. Hungary has an entirely integrated national bloodtransfusion service. There are 24 larger and 40 smaller bloodtransfusion centres professionally directed and supervised by the National Institute of Haematology and Blood Transfusion (NIHBT), which is the basic institution for haematology, immunology and bloodtransfusion of the Ministry of Health. The institute has in-patient and out-patient departments for patients with haematological and immunological diseases, all the departments for the collection, processing and distribution of a broad spectrum of blood components and plasma derivatives. It is also an institute for basic and applied research in haematology, immunology and bloodtransfusion. From budgetary and personnel point of view the regional centres function as departments of teaching hospitals, county- and city hospitals, which means that they are also fully integrated into the country's national health service. The high degree of decentralization of the bloodtransfusion service was aimed at achieving a nation-wide improvement in the clinical use of blood and blood derivatives, and the availability of high level treatment of patients with haematological diseases in every part of the country.

Every two months a two-days postgraduate education course on selected topics of recent advances in haematology, immunology and bloodtransfusion is held for the directors of the regional centres at the NIHBT. Before the application of a new method in routine work of our national blood service, heads of departments and technicians from each regional centre are trained in the NIHBT. On the other hand the directors and the professional staff members of the regional centres give postgraduate teaching sessions to physicians and surgeons of the region which they supply with blood and blood components. This enables us to teach 700 doctors yearly by regular postgraduate courses. In every field of clinical medicine where bloodtransfusions are being administered routinely, doctors have to attend a two-weeks postgraduate course in bloodtransfusion before they are accepted to sit for an examination for the degree of their special field i.e. anaesthesiology, surgery, traumatology, medicine, paediatrics, obstetrics and gynaecology. Every young physician has to attend a five-days course on "Basic principles of bloodtransfusion in clinical practice" before being accepted as a resident. We find this essential because it is reasonable to expect that the physician responsible for prescribing blood and blood derivatives has an understanding of how it is provided, and when and how to use it safely and efficiently.

The fact that the directors of bloodtransfusion centres in Hungary can achieve some basic clinical practice and training in haematology and immunology enables them to give high-level postgraduate courses to clinicians of their region. This is the key to building up a close liaison with clinical units. As a result clinicians consult our experts and we can fight efficiently against the misuse of blood. The results are much better than those which can be achieved by autocratic measures. The efficiency of the postgraduate teaching program is well reflected in the region by the improved use of cell concentrates instead of whole blood. According to our experience the new level is being sustained for approximately six to twelve months. Consequently, the battle against the misuse of whole blood cannot be won by a single postgraduate course or with a symposium on the optimal use of blood. Postgraduate training courses have to be repeated regularly and should always include the most recent results to attract the attention of the participants.

The programs of postgraduate treaching of residents and senior staff do not include detailes of scientific and technological matters of processing of blood components and plasma fractions, or other basic functions of bloodtransfusion centres. Most of the time is devoted to clinical uses and misuses of bloodtransfusion in the context of modern clinical medicine. It is stressed throughout the educational program that every patient represents an individual case and consequently no standard prescriptions but only scientifically based recommendations can be given. In final analysis the trainee must apply the available information to the solution of patient care problems. Safety aspects of the clinical use of blood and derivatives represent core subjects of the training.

National education programs have to be revised regularly to include the most recent advances and internationally evaluated and accepted new principles and methods in bloodtransfusion practice. The ongoing sharing of information and technology, the elaboration of international standards and recommendations for products and methods are of utmost importance in this rapidly advancing field of medicine. It is also a continuous endeavour of the World Health Organization, the League of Red Cross Societies and the International Society of Blood Transfusion to join all efforts to achieve optimal and safe use of blood not only at a national but also at an international level.

DISCUSSION

Moderators: Ch.L. Sonnenberg, J.A. van der Does

H.F. Taswell, Rochester, USA:

Mr. van der Meulen, the job description that you use and the whole process of job analysis and planning as you so well describe is a very clear tool for quality assurance and quality control. You mentioned in passing the importance of choosing the right number of people, and the related question of future planning. I wonder if you could take just a few minutes to discuss methods of choosing the correct number and how that is related to future planning.

H. van der Meulen, Groningen, The Netherlands:

It is difficult to talk about future developments. It means we should try to get an idea of future developments within the requirements for the jobs. It probably can be done by techniques such as ratio analysis and the conduct of brainstorming sessions.

H.F. Taswell:

In respect to the very first question, I was thinking of the practice of what we refer to as workload recording, which we have been working with for the last four or five years. I find this an extremely valuable management tool as well as a quality control tool. Because it does not help to have selected the right person and written a good job description, and provide the proper equipment and reagents, and then have them so overworked that they cannot do their job, or so underworked that they get into trouble. So, one has to choose the right number. This can be done, I am convinced, in a very objective manner with properly trained people using a stopwatch. Most procedures in blood banking are very amenable to this kind of approach. Each procedure, whether it is compatibility testing or collecting a unit of blood, can be timed and one can figure out exactly what fixed time and what variable time each procedure takes, multiply by the number of activities that are going on, and calculate quite accurately just how many people are needed for that particular activity. Then, observing the increase of activity by year, it becomes quite easy to do future planning. It also makes it very easy to justify requests for additional employees. It is very hard to argue with that kind of numbers. We found this to be a very effective tool.

W.L. Marsh, New York, USA:

Can I ask Dr. Hollán: What kind of procedure do you have in the training and the selection of eventual medical directors for your regional blood selection blood centres?

S.R. Hollán, Budapest, Hungary:

The main principle is that we want to have physicians and not surgeons as directors. We want them to have some clinical experience. They have to have, of course, intensive individual training. We have a degree for specialization in bloodtransfusion in Hungary. This is awarded after a three-year training. One of these years must be spent in the National Institute of Haematology. At least one year must be spent in a large regional centre. The remaining year can be spent in any other centre. We take into consideration whether they have spent time in a clinical department. We also look for good organizers and motivated persons. It is important that they have the right personality, from the standpoint of approaching people. The transfusion centre cannot function efficiently if the director does not establish good contacts with key persons in the region, as well as with the regular blood donors. These are the main principles.

W.L. Marsh:

Do I understand that this is a specific program aimed at directors? In the New York Blood Center and other parts of America, we have specific programs. For example, we have a blood bank director's program. This is a program in which we take young doctors that wish to specialize in the field and become directors of blood banks. We train them very specifically with this end in mind. Your program is in effect doing the same thing: selecting people whose ambition and aim is to be a director of a blood centre.

C.Th. Smit Sibinga, Groningen, The Netherlands:

Did I understand correctly that the basic philosophy and the approach which Dr. Myhre has listed in his presentation is more a type of competency-oriented training extending to the selection of personnel or is it a type of further educational training of personnel once you are sure to have recruited the right competent people?

A second question is: Is the system which you apply an integral one, is your senior staff involved in the final training, or do you have a separate department in your centre which is fully dedicated to this type of education, i.e. designing the program, evaluating the program talking to people?

B.A. Myhre, Torrance, USA:

In my own specific hospital I do have two registrars assigned to me at any one time. We will have in addition to that some new technologists. We have been very fortunate in not having had a larger turnover, so that we have not had to train too many new ones. We have a clinical technology school from which we do have two to four students assigned to the blood bank all the time. The residents change every three months, the medical technology students change monthly. So, over a period of a year between 20 and 40 medical technology students will have gone through the program.

Each of these basically go through a semi-rigid training program. By the time they are through, they must have satisfied the various categories. Let me take my registrars as an example: daily they are expected to make rounds and find out what is going on in the service. This is done between 8 and 9 a.m. We meet at nine o'clock and discuss any cases that are to be handled, that are problems. If we feel that those patients need to be visited, we will visit.

Over the period of three months, we will go through a curriculum of training for these two people. By the time they are through, I will have been able to check off that they were exposed to all aspects. As some of you know, I have a hobby of computer-assisted education. Therefore, by the time they are through, they will have taken a test in every blood group system on the computer. At the end, they are strongly encouraged to take the Proficiency Testing Examination, which is given by the American Society of Clinical Pathology. This examination is unique in the fact that there is a booklet with it that explains each of the answers. So by the time we are through, we have gone through a program. It is not a formal program as such. I actually used to show slides and give canned lectures. I found we all got bored. So, now we do have topics for each week. We rotate so that each of the registrars presents one day and I take the third day; or, if it is in an area I particularly like I will do it anyway. In addition to that, if there is a patient with an unique problem, we may talk about that patient that day.

Our medical technology program runs somewhat the same, except there we have them for a month, then they are gone. At the end of the year, they will be taking their licensing examination. Therfore, they are under the control of one of our technologists, who does most of the training. She will go ahead and make certain that each of the categories are satisfied, so that they are ready for their registry examination at the end of that time.

C.Th. Smit Sibinga:

So, this type of education you are providing is a type of undergraduate education. You make different aspects of bloodtransfusion an integral part of other training programs, for instance internal medicine, or medical technology. The students are trained in aspects of bloodtransfusion and leave the blood bank and go their way. Once they apply for a job – and this is what Mr. van der Meulen was trying to convey to us as a message – they already have had some training in bloodtransfusion aspects.

A question to Dr. Hollán with regard to her beautiful program in Hungary. We were not aware of this, but should you not start it one step back in education? Should we not more actively integrate bloodtransfusion as a type of clinical science in the medical education of our students, in stead of waiting untill graduation, to make them aware of what blood actually is and what it can do?

S.R. Hollán:

It is a very good question. In fact I have mentioned too, that it is most surprising that medical students do not get a systematic theoretical basis and practice in bloodtransfusion. Why we do not do this is for the following reason: the medical training of students is so "overjammed" that there is a continuous struggle between the various subjects for more education. I share the opinion of those who suggest that medical schools, should aim to educate well-trained practitioners, since most of the students have to enter this type of jobs. This is why I think that for the present clinical haematology and bloodtransfusion as special subjects for specialization should be taught in depth in post-graduate teaching.

H.F. Taswell:

Dr. Hollán, of the two parts of the training program that we talked about, Dr. Myhre talked about initial training. One aspect of that is quite easy, since we have a captive audience and we can give them the training that is necessary. For the other part, continuing education, the problem is that those who need it most are not always there to receive it. How do you approach that problem?

You listed a large number of people to whom you give continuous education: donors, clinicians, blood bank employees and so on. The blood bank employee is a little easier to reach for a continuing training program. How do you get the clinicians to come for the continuing training programs?

S.R. Hollán:

I want to stress that the continuous education program for the professional house staff is done regularly, and they have to teach what they have learned to the clinicians in their region. This gives good results. It is no problem to encourage physicians and surgeons to participate in the postgraduate courses of bloodtransfusion, haematology, immunology, since they cannot obtain a degree in their specialization without following these courses. However, it is much more difficult to get the senior staff, i.e. the professors.

By holding consultations and really getting down to the discussion of problems, we feel that we can deal with heads of departments, keeping them informed about recent advances in haemotherapy.

B.A. Myhre:

I realize that I have really not answered Dr. Smit Sibinga's question completely. What do you do with a new employee? Some of them may be very well trained and some may be very poorly trained. We treat a new employee basically the same way we do a student. The new employees come in and are exposed to the same set of lectures as the students are, except it may take five minutes to give them the lecture once we realize that they know the area, where it takes an hour for the student. They have to demonstrate their proficiency in the same way. As to the students, they have to pass the same kind of examination. This is kept on record, so that later if somebody says in a court of law: "Was this person competent?" we can say: "Yes, they went through this training program; they passed this examination, and so forth". So, we go through all those things the same way, except we do expect a higher level of performance from a working technologist than we do from a student. In addition to that, we do have continuing education programs in which a topic is brought up weekly for all our staff. The other thing Dr. Taswell was talking about, which I fully agree on, and in our case is an absolute necessity, is the use of the American College of Pathologists Workload Recording System. This very nicely gives you a weighing for every test you do. In every shift you work out how many tests were done and the total units, devide them by the number of employee hours and come up with a productivity index. Currently, our productivity index is running at 45, which represents 45 minutes out of every hour a person is supposed to be working at some test, which is considered about right. If I had, right now, a productivity index of 45 and tried to go to my administrator to get more help, I can forget it. On the other hand, if it begins to go up to 55 or 60, I have a good justification for getting personnel. If it is down to 30, I am in big trouble. So, it makes it a very nice method. The only way to deviate from that is by offering new procedures. Then these can be rated again by means of the Workload Recording Index, to estimate how many people you will need.

C.Th. Smit Sibinga:

It is extremely important, as stated by Mrs. Sonnenberg at the opening of this session, that there is hardly any real attention paid to the personnel aspect, particularly at the blood banks. Blood banks are still regarded in many places in the world as a type of backdoor medicine practice, something you can learn on a Friday afternoon. This is no longer the case today. Bloodtransfusion is a very complicated aspect of clinical medicine, as we deal with a living tissue, a transplant. Therefore, what we learn from these presentations is that we should go back and sit down, and try to find ways to make protocols and procedures for these aspects. In the USA there is a system already in application for years in which postgraduates have to catch up with the state of the art and new developments, in a credit-point type of system. This is a system which obliges people to come and collect the credit points.

Ch.L. Sonnenberg, Rochester, USA:

Many of our organizations around the country, not only blood banking, but medical technology organizations and special areas such as microbiology, are beginning to have a system where all of the members are required to have a certain number of continuing-education credits every year. Therefore, it is compulsory to go to these continuing-education meetings. It forces people to present papers and to attend good quality programs, because there are certain criteria necessary in order to get acceptable credits. It forces individuals to take the responsibility of their continuing education upon themselves. We are seeing that more and more frequently. I think it is a good thing.

R.J. Crawford, Glasgow, Scotland:

Talking about continuing education. Our licensing body in the UK is now suggesting that we should do internal proficiency tests of all matching staff at frequent intervals, and add that to the documentation of the employee record. It is an instrument in the event someone makes a mistake and possibly harms a patient. It provides two ways forwards. One is, you can say to the Procurator Fiscal: "Here is the documentary evidence that this man was thought to be competent to do the job that we left him to do". The second thing you can do with the record is to show it to the employee and say: "We are very sorry you killed that patient, but this is the evidence which led us to have confidence in you and which means that we still have confidence in you, even in spite of this deplorable accident". So, I think records and proficiency testing are an internal medium of continuing education. After that, in the proficiency testing you can force the on-call technician to interpret hideous results instead of test sera and make him decide when he should call a doctor.

Ch.L. Sonnenberg:

I defenitely agree. One of the important things in proficiency testing whether external or internal, is that these testings should be performed by the people actually doing the work. I know of situations in which it was the supervisor who always performed the proficiency tests to be sure to get the answer correct. This is not appropriate. What we want to do is find out what the people are doing, how are they doing. The ones that are working at the bench, are the important individuals. You should keep that in mind with proficiency testing.

P. Rebulla, Milan, Italy:

What is the actual type of examination given to people who are training in institutions? Is it written, is it practical? What are the problems they have to face? Can they talk to the people in the blood bank regularly?

B.A. Myhre:

We use a combination. We give practical examinations in which they are given specimens to determine. We give multiple choice examinations and oral interviews.

S.R. Hollán:

Those who pass a number of training courses have to do practical examinations in different departments of the National Institute of Haematology and Blood Transfusion. They have to perform the most important tests and the most important production methods and get a mark first for their practical training. After this, they will sit for an oral examination. We have a type of examination for postgraduate courses lasting two or three weeks. This is composed of multiple choice examinations and oral interviews. Of course, we also have practical tests in serology.

H. van der Meulen:

I am not teaching any blood bank people or university students, but there is a growing tendency in the universities to use multiple choice tests. There are some disadvantages to this system, as it only serves to produce a recollection of facts. I much prefer an oral test, which would reveal whether they know the "inside" of the matter. I would advocate also practical examinations.

C.F. Högman, Uppsala, Sweden:

According to my experience, one of the most difficult things to teach people is to make them understand how easy it is to make mistakes. For such reason, I think it is important to devise some type of exercise to demonstrate this. We have done this by simply letting the students doe testings on unknown samples. This type of exercise is important, because they believe they cannot make mistakes. Unfortunately, it frequently turns out that there is a high incidence of mistakes in, for instance, ABO type, or Rhesus. According to our experience, more mistakes are made in Rh than in ABO typing.

H.F. Taswell:

Cheryl Sonnenberg is assigned the task of teaching all new employees and medical students, physicians, residents, or trainees; everyone who has been through our blood bank for the last ten years. She has done a very, very excellent job. In our institution we have an election every year in which a teacher is nominated for a Great Teacher's Award. Cheryl is the recipient of such an award. Perhaps she will say a few words about education in the blood bank.

Ch.L. Sonnenberg:

When I first began teaching, I had no background in teaching. I was trained as a medical technologist. It took me a few years to get my facts together. But I did learn a few things that may be helpful to you. One of the things that I learned was that each individual is different. A very structured, organized program that each individual must follow on a certain timetable, does not work. This is something you have to keep in mind. I found that we had such a variety of students that one specific program, as Dr. Myhre said, is not workable for every type of student. So, I categorized students, just as Dr. Myhre did, which is an essential point in any educational program: the categorization of a blood bank director trainee versus a clinical pathology resident, a haematology resident, a specialist in blood banking coming to work in your blood bank or a medical technology student. Each individual is different. I began by writing goals and objectives. It is extremely important to know what you want your student to be able to do. So, objectives are extremely important. The objectives may be similar for each student group, or they may be different. They may be more intense for a particular group, while you might just want to give the basic facts to another group. Rather than have a matrix like Dr. Myhre, we have what we call check lists where we actually list out for each type of student the items that we want them to learn. And, we chek it off as they have learned. With established objectives you have the means of evaluating whether or not your student has accomplished that objective. So, you want to know what the student will be able to do, and then you want to know: Has he accomplished that objective. In a nutshell, that is basically our educational program.

IV. Clinical efficacy

TRANSFUSION PRACTICE: ASPECTS OF SAFETY RELATED TO CLINICAL EFFICACY

H. de Beus, C.Th. Smit Sibinga

INTRODUCTION

To obtain a maximum degree of quality of blood and blood components in order to assure the highest level of safety in everyday's transfusion practice, a complexity of actions is necessary.

According to WHO (1) these actions should relate to the safety, purity, potency and clinical efficacy of the final blood components, where the clinician takes full responsibility for bloodtransfusion practice at the bed-side.

Amongst these actions are to be named:

a. all the safety precautions in collecting the donor blood;
b. all the administrative procedures which conduct the collecting and processing of the blood;
c. the obligatory and necessary laboratory control;
d. all the specific quality control, safeguarding the production of the different blood components.

This complexity of actions all together is called "Good Manufacturing Practice" (GMP). GMP not only covers the necessary control of the standard to be achieved, but more important leads to the assurance of quality to the medical consumer.

To ensure optimal clinical efficacy, GMP should be followed by an identical process inside the hospital, at the bed-side. This in-hospital complexity of actions is called "Good Hospital Practice" (GHP). Basically GMP and GHP should be regarded as twin brother and sister, closely related to and depending on each other. Although GMP is fully accepted, and practiced in most blood banks, GHP still is not regarded as an essential part of all day routine hospital practice. This particularly applies to bloodtransfusion practice, which in general lacks the dedication it deserves!

There are several reasons for this phenomenon, none of them being an excuse:

a. The people working on the GMP side are all full time employees in their job, where the average clinician spends only a minor part of his time on bloodtransfusion. Routine workloads on the average seem to have more priorities than just bloodtransfusion.

b. Although in the laboratory practice GMP is relatively young, the workers are specifically trained as professionals. The average clinician using the blood bank range of products hardly ever is specifically educated and trained in the GHP standard of infusion and transfusion practice. Even the anaesthesiologist, being the medical specialist who spends a substantial amount of his routine working time on infusion and transfusion practice, experiences that the specific knowledge and expertise related to transfusion practice so far is gained almost exclusively after being graduated. GHP seems to be carreer bound in stead of a fundamental of medical education.

Summarizing the introduction it can be stated that:

a. The clinical specialist is the final link in the chain of events of quality assurance in bloodtransfusion from donor to patient.
b. He cannot practice blood transfusion according to the highest standard unless he accepts the rules of GHP as the only guideline in achieving an optimal efficacy of bloodtransfusion.
c. Quality assurance in clinical transfusion practice in the first place is a mental attitude, a process of critical self control.

PRACTICAL ASPECTS

For good standard practice in bloodtransfusion an optimal choice of the technical equipment, the outfit, is necessary. This means the evaluation of knowledge and expertise to ensure the highest level of quality of the different tools needed for transfusion practice.

The clinician has to reflect on the specific requirements for each part of the total infusion or transfusion software chain:

1. the intravenous cannula;
2. the administration set;
3. the container;

and in addition to the main chain:

1. pressure cuffs;
2. infusion pumps;
3. bloodwarming apparatus;
4. micro-filters.

Apart from these specific technical aspects it is even more important to realise how to use these materials:

a. where and how to perform the phlebotomy;
b. how to prevent local infection – in situ period of intravenous cannula, period of usage of administration set.

From the clinical point of view one can distinguish two fields of practice, belonging to GHP:

1. laboratory practice, which is extensively dealt with in other papers;
2. clinical transfusion practice.

It is clear that a critical attitude towards the standard bloodtransfusion policy as developed by each physician during his practice, can yield a remarkable reduction in the overusage of blood and blood components.

In clinical transfusion practice the following questions are of essential importance:

a. is there any need for blood transfusion?
b. when there is a need, what then is the specific indication and what blood component is needed?
c. how many units have to be transfused?
d. how to give these units practically?

In this presentation we will exclusively deal with the last question, the bed-side technique of transfusion practice. In general, the absence of information about this aspect of transfusion practice inside the hospital is remarkable and astonishing. Even Mollison (2) in his famous textbook "Blood Transfusion in Clinical Practice" does not spend a single page on the subject. Neither does the latest WHO publication (3) about "The Collection, Fractionation, Quality Control and Uses of Blood and Blood Products"!

So far only the American Association of Blood Banks dedicates a separate chapter to clinical practice in recent publications like "Guidelines to Transfusion Practice" 1980 (4) and "Safe Transfusion" 1981 (5). For a good bed-side technique in transfusion practice, choice of material and equipment, the different parts of the infusion or transfusion chain, is essential. As mentioned before, this transfusion chain always consists of three parts: the container, the administration set and the intravenous cannula.

Essential requirements for the infusion or transfusion chain are:

a. it should be a closed system;
b. it should be disconnection proof, in other words the integrety of the infusion chain is of major importance in quality assurance.

Both requirements are primarily factors in defining the risks of extrinsic contamination. Every clinical specialist should be aware of the fact that the incidence of intrinsic or manufacturer defined contamination is extremely low thanks to GMP. On the other hand the overall incidence of extrinsic or in-use contamination is relatively high. According to Maki (6) about 5% of all in-use transfusion chains must be considered to be contaminated, almost all of them iatrogenic and therefore preventable!

Blood and blood products are from a bacteriological point of view very vulnerable fluids, providing favourable growing conditions to most of the micro-organisms which accidentally invade the transfusion system. This is mostly due to a lack of care and dedication of those responsible for bed-side transfusion practice.

A. The container. Blood banks almost exclusively collect, process and issue blood and blood components in closed systems, P.V.C. non-vented bags. In this respect transfusion practice is far ahead infusion practice. In many hospitals still glass bottles are in use for infusion fluids. Primarily for bacteriolgical reasons these should be abandoned from clinical practice.

B. The administration set (AS). Based on the criteria as given for the transfusion chain, being a closed and disconnection proof system, the criteria for an optimal AS are:

1. spike – to ensure an optimal connection to a P.V.C. bag.
2. a luer lock connector to ensure the disconnection proof principle on the intervenous cannula side.
3. filter house, providing a filter chamber with a 150-170 μ pore-size mesh filter in the upper part and a dripping chamber in the lower part of the filter house. For transfusion of any blood component whether cells or plasma proteins, such a mesh filter is mandatory.
4. Y type of AS, a filter house with two container connection lines should be the system of choice for transfusion of blood and blood components. It provides the possibility for priming and rinsing by a separate saline connected line, where this can be used as well for diluting the red cell concentrate to decrease the viscosity by addition of 0.9% saline.
5. the length of the AS is not a major criterium for selection. In general an AS shorter than a 150 cm is highly impracticable, whereas a length greater than 250 cm also causes trouble. As an optimum, 200 cm ± 10 seems to be the best.

C. Intravenous cannula. In the older days the selection of intravenous cannulae was restricted to two types of Vanadium steel needles. The plastic industry has caused a major and universal break through in the field of intravenous cannula, starting with P.V.C., polypropylene and polyethylene catheters, where nowadays almost exclusively teflon type of cannula are being manufactured in a wide variety. Today 1982 there are over 18 types of cannulae available on the Dutch market. For a proper selection there can be distinguished at least eight different criteria as there are boresize, material, colour-coded conus, locking system, bavel indication etc.

Most of the cannula available do differ in any respects, with the sole exception of all having a luer lock connection to the administration system. Apart from the careful selection procedure of the best tool for phlebotomy, a more important question arises: How to handle the intravenous cannula.

Even the best instrument may lead to bad results when handled wrongly! In this respect the following points are of importance:

1. where to place the intravenous cannula;
2. which precautions should be taken to prevent infection from the point of entrance of the intravenous cannula;
3. which priming solution is needed;
4. what is the maximum acceptable in-situ period of the intravenous cannula;
5. how long a period of time can the administration set be used in line;
6. identification of the patient and the product to be transfused – administrative and physical control;
7. is addition of drugs to the transfusion chain allowable;
8. control of patient's reactions to the transfusion – temperature, blood pressure, pulse rate and respiration, allergic phenomena, in order to detect and document an adverse reaction.

It will be clear that all of these points, apart from specific aspects like osmolarity and acidity of the infusion fluid alternatively given, are of great importance for the risks of thrombophlebitis or even septichaemia in the course of infusion or transfusion therapy. Therefor these eight points will be discussed individually.

Ad 1. From the literature there is no consensus to be distilled as to decide where to insert the intravenous cannula. Thomas (1970) (7) could not find a significant relation between phlebitis and the location of the cannula, where he tested the back of the hand, the wrist, the fore-arm and the elbow. In contrast Müller (1972) (8) did find a relation between thrombophlebitis and the site of insertion.

The incidence of phlebitis did increase significantly from proximal to distal - elbow 11.5%, fore-arm 21.2%, hand 31.6%. There is more than one reason for these differences, a mechanical factor being one of the conditions of the high incidence of phlebitis on the back of the hand. An additional point seems to be the necessity for a high blood flow, especially important where hypertonic and/or acidic infusion solutions are being used. The fore-arm seems to be the most acceptable site both for the comfort of the patient, the possibilities for fixing the cannula as well as the guarantee of a patent and continuous flow of the infusion or transfusion.

Ad 2. Infection prevention during phlebotomy is not always taken serious. Nevertheless, a plea has to be made for a high standard of aseptic phlebotomy, followed by an aseptic regime on the ward. It is generally agreed that part of the post-infusion thrombophlebitis problem is caused by skin commensal flora of the patient himself, like Staphylococcus albus and Streptococcus epidermidis and even occasionally Enterococcae. Smallman et. al. (1980) (11) did a comparitive study on the effect of skin preparation and care on the incidence of superficial thrombophlebitis between two groups of patients, one group without and the second group with a regime of antiseptic skin preparation. In the first group 100% of the patients developed a superficial thrombophlebitis after 2.4 days, whereas only 24.5% of patients from the antiseptic group developed the same complication. The following rules should be standard in transfusion practice:

1. handwashing (desinfection) of the phlebotomist;
2. shaving of the patient's skin;
3. intensive swabbing with a desinfectant for example povidone-iodine or chlorohexidine;
4. aseptic covering of the phlebotomy wound with a gauze dipped in for instance providone-iodine ointment and fixation of the cannula with plasters.

This point can very well be summarized quoting Maki et. al. (1973) (12): "The cannula site is not unlike an open surgical wound containing a foreign body. The insertion of a catheter should be considered a minor surgical procedure, ...".

Ad 3. Priming solution (compatibility). Normal saline (0.9% NaCl) has been the ideal solution for priming an AS from the very first days of transfusion practice on. It is the only solution which is compatible to blood and neither causes hemolysis nor clumping of red cells or clotting of the blood (9). In contrast to this, Ringer's and Hartman's solution as well as 5% dextrose are absolutely contra-indicated. Dextrose causes red cell clumping and also a rapid haemolysis of red cells. Both the Ringer's and Hartman's solution contain enough ionized calcium to overcome the anticoagulant effect of citrate, allowing small clots to develop in the transfusion chain. As to other solutions different opinions can be read from the literature. Ryden and Oberman (10) studied both the combination of 0.45% saline/2.5% dextrose as well as 0.4% saline/5% dextrose. In their study no red cell damaging effect was noticed, although the use of these solutions does not give any benefit over normal saline.

Ad 4. In-situ period of the intravenous cannula. In the last decade a great number of publications concerning the importance of the length of time the intravenous cannula is left in the vein related to the incidence of thrombophlebitis has been published. In 1972 the Center for Disease Control (CDC) (15) has advised the following: "Indwelling cannula should not be left in place longer than 72 hours, and preferably be changed at 48 hours interval". The CDC also recommends to change the AS every 24 hours and in any event every time the intravenous cannula is changed.

Altemeyer et. al. (1971) (16) based on what they called "The third day surgical fever", advised to change AS and cannula every 48 hours. Since then an ever growing number of publications point to even shorter periods, for instance 24 hours. Thomas et. al. (7) wrote in their classical paper (1970) "The severity of local complications was directly related to the mean infusion time". There was a direct correlation between the duration of the infusion and the incidence of infectious complications. During the first 24 hours the relationship was linear and highly significant. Dinley (17) describes the steady increase in the number of infectious reactions seen during the initial 24 hours period for all cannulae and to a slightly lesser extent during subsequent periods of 24 hours. He, too, reported a statistically highly significant difference in the number of infectious complications between patients receiving bloodtransfusion and patients treated with standard infusion fluid regimes (Table I). The significant difference was noted after 24 as well as 48 hours period of infusion. Based on the many observations and well documented studies it becomes evident that for a GHP only the shortest in-situ period is acceptable. One should change the cannula and the AS before venous complications develop and not, as is often seen on ward rounds, after the infection became manifest!

In our hospital we agree on a practical compromise: Maximal 48 hours, unless the patient has no real alternative due to lack of venous access. In the latter case a choice has to be made between:

1. heparin prophylaxis;
2. venesection and heparin prophylaxis;
3. vena cava catheter (vena jugularis interna or vena subclavia)

The latter choice should be regarded as an ultimum refugium because of the high risk of infections and other complications from this type of catheters.

Tabel I. Incidence of venous complications with the addition of blood to the intravenous infusion, over 24 and 48 hour periods: all cannulae.

Time period	Total infusions	Blood infusions	%	Significant
24 hours	197	38	19.3	
No complications	107	3	2.8	p < 0.01
Venous complications	90	35	38.9	
48 hours	418	122	29.2	
No complications	177	3	1.7	p < 0.001
Venous complications	241	119	49.4	

From: Dingley, R.J., Curr. Med. Res. and Opinion 9:607, 1976.

Ad 5. Period of use of AS. With respect to the change of AS policy, the CDC (1972) (15) advised to change every 24 hours. This very vigorous advice has to be seen against the background of the tremendous misery many American hospitals went through after the greatest explosion of intrinsic contamination of intravenous therapy, the so-called Abbott affaire 1970–1971. Before that time, a routine change of AS at periodic intervals was not practiced. The same AS was used for the total duration of infusion therapy or until malfunction (Maki 1976) (18). Since the disaster, a policy of replacing AS every 24 hours has become an accepted practice at approximately 80% of hospitals in the USA (CDC) (19). However, in the late seventies several papers were published in order to analyse the need and also the cost effectiveness of this policy. Band and Maki (20) observed that the incidence of infusion phlebitis when the AS was changed after 48 hours did not differ from a change every 24 hours. It was concluded that: "Based on the findings of this study ... adapting 48 hours as the interval for routine change of delivery systems, seems justified in terms of safety and could result in considerable savings to hospitals".

However, three situations as exceptions using the 48 hrs interval were distinguished:

a. after administration of blood products;
b. after administration of fat emulsions;
c. when an epidemic of infusion related septicaemia is suspected.

In these cases the 24 hours interval should be adopted again. Buxton et. al. (1979) (21) compared the rates of intravenous associated bacteremia in 2 series of 300 patients, one changed at 24 hours interval and the other at 48 hours interval. Both groups had comparable rates of phlebitis. There was no advantage from changing the AS every 24 hours over every 48 hours. Taking all these studies into consideration the following can be recommended:

1. routine interval for changing AS: 48 hours;
2. in case of bloodtransfusion or infusion of fat emulsions or in case of suspected infusion related infection: change immediately and do not wait till the 24 hours period has expired.

Where most of the extrinsic contaminations are likely to occur during manipulation of the infusion or transfusion chain, therefor restrict the 48 hours interval to the routine ward patients, but maintain the 24 hours interval for all patients on intensive or coronary care units.

Ad 6. Patient–product identification. In the totality of quality assurance measures according to GHP, this aspect is of critical importance. Although bloodtransfusion has become a routine and rather safe type of medical treatment, there still exists a mortality due to transfusion therapy. Myhre (13), in analyzing a 113 deaths resulting from blood transfusion between 1976 and 1979 reported to FDA, concluded that almost two thirds of the fatal reactions were related to misidentification of the patient, the blood sample or the unit of blood administered. The most common error was administration of a unit of blood to the wrong patient! Over 50% of the deaths in this series could easily have been prevented. The results of this study can only have one consequence: The moral and legal obligation for all workers in laboratory and clinical practice of bloodtransfusion to check and double check. Never rely on administrative information. A manual of GHP with written rules and regulations should be mandatory in every hospital. The transfusionist, whether nurse or doctor self-evidently has to practice according to these rules and regulations. To quote Grilli (1981) (14): "The best guarantee of safe transfusion is strict adherence to policy and procedures".

Ad 7. Addition of drugs. The addition of drugs of any kind to blood or blood components results in protein binding of the drug and therefor in many cases inactivation, the formation of immunogenic complexes, adhesion of drugs on red cell membranes and other non-wanted effects. When drugs have to be administered intravenously they should be given directly intravenously and not injected in any part of the transfusion chain. The AABB in its Standard for Blood Banks and Transfusion Services (22) states very clearly: "No drugs should be added to blood or blood components".

Ad 8. Controlling patients' reactions to transfusion. As bloodtransfusion in clinical practice is the transplantation of a living human tissue, this transplant practice should be very carefully monitored. Especially immediate phenomena of incompatibility or rejection, the so-called transfusion reactions, should be monitored, controlled and documented with great accuracy. As an integral part of GHP it is the responsibility of the nurse and the doctor to carefully monitor, control and document every transfusion of blood or blood components.

CONCLUSION

The totality of precautions and actions, rules and regulations with respect to everyday routine transfusion practice comprises what we now call GHP. The main and ultimate aim of GHP is to assure a maximum safety of the patient receiving blood transfusion. Without the continuing care and dedication of particularly an infusion/transfusion committee and every individual transfusionist such a practice can never be achieved. Every hospital needs to have a transfusion committee to ensure quality in bed-side transfusion practice. The main functions of such a committee can be defined as:

1. advising and supervising;
2. writing and updating an infusion/transfusion manual;
3. controlling the standard practice to assure the highest level of quality in bloodtransfusion practice.

Salus aegroti suprema lex!

REFERENCES

1. WHO, Technical Series 626, Geneva, 1978.
2. Mollison, P.L. Blood transfusion in clinical medicine. 6th ed. Oxford: Blackwell Scientific Publ., 1979.
3. WHO. The collection, fractionation, quality control and uses of blood and blood products. Geneva, 1980.
4. Guidelines to transfusion practices. American Association of Blood Banks, Washington, DC, 1980.
5. Safe transfusion. American Association of Blood Banks, Washington, DC, 1981.
6. Maki, D.G. Sepsis arising from extrinsic contamination of the infusion and measures for control. In: Philips, I., Meers, P.D., D'Arcy, P.F. (eds.) Microbiological hazards of infusion therapy, 1976, pp. 99–143.
7. Thomas, E.T., Evers, W., Gabor, B.R. Postinfusion phlebitis. Anaesth. & Analgesia Curr. Res. 1970;1:150–9.
8. Müller, C., Koch, P., Schakriari, S. Bakteriologische Nachuntersuchungen bei Cava Kathetern. Z.Prakt. Anaesth. 1972; 7:55–60.
9. Technical Manual. 7th ed. American Association of Blood Banks, Washington, DC, 1977.
10. Ryder, S.E., Oberman, H.A. Compatibility of common intravenous solutions with CPD blood. Transfusion 1975;15:250–5.
11. Smallman, L., Burdon, D.W., Williams, J.A. The effect of skin preparation and care on the incidence of superficial thrombophlebitis. Birt. J. Surg. 1980;67:861–2.
12. Maki, D.G., Goldman, D.A, Rhame, F.S. Infection control in intravenous therapy. Ann. Int. Med. 1973;79:867–87.
13. Myhre, B.A. Fatalities from blood transfusion. JAMA 1980;244: 1333–5.

14. Grilli, E. Technical aspects of transfusion. In: Safe transfusion. American Association of Blood Banks, Washington, DC, 1981, pp. 47–62.
15. Center for Disease Control. Training bulletin hospital infection and microbiological control sections. Bacterial disease, branches epidemiology Program, 1972.
16. Altemeyer, W.A., McDonough, J.J., Fullen, W.D. Third day surgical fever. Arch. Surg. 1971;103:158–66.
17. Dinley, R.J. Venous reactions related to in-dwelling plastic cannulae. A prospective clinical trial. Curr. Med. Res. Opin. 1976;3:607–17.
18. Maki, D.G., Rhame, F.S., Mackel, D.C., Bennett, J.V. Nationwide epidemic of septicemia caused by contaminated intravenous products. I: Epidemiologic and clinical features. Am. J. Med. 1976;80:471–80.
19. Center for Disease Control. Infection, surveillance and control programs in US hospitals. An assessment. Morbid Mortal Weekly Rep. 1978;27:139–45.
20. Band, J.D., Maki, D.G. Safety of changing intravenous delivery systems at longer than 24 hours interval. Ann. Int. Med. 1979;91: 173–8.
21. Buxton, A.E., Highsmith, A.K., Garner, J.S. et. al. Contamination of intravenous infusion fluid: effects of changing administration sets. Ann. Int. Med. 1979;90:764–8.
22. Standards for Blood Banks and Transfusion Services. 11th ed. American Association of Blood Banks, Washington, DC, 1981.

TRANSFUSION REACTIONS

K. Sintnicolaas

INTRODUCTION

The transfusion of blood and its components is a widely used form of supportive therapy and this field has expanded greatly in recent years due to the development of more intensive treatment modalities. This is particularly true for patients with malignant diseases, where the application of high dose cytotoxic therapy often results in periods of severe bone marrow depression. This has stimulated the development of a sophisticated platelet and granulocyte substitution therapy. However, we must bear in mind that a significant number of transfusions are complicated by adverse effects and in fact patients still die from fatal transfusion reactions.

This paper will deal with these adverse effects, in particular with the immune-mediated reactions, of which there are two types:

- those occurring during or immediately following transfusion – the immediate reactions, and
- those with a time interval of several days between transfusion and reaction – the delayed-type reactions.

Hemolytic, febrile and allergic transfusion reactions are immediate reactions, as is non-cardiogenic pulmonary edema. Hemolysis may also appear as a delayed-type reaction. Other delayed-type reactions are graft-versus-host disease, posttransfusion purpura and the development of alloimmunization to blood cell antigens.

HEMOLYTIC TRANSFUSION REACTIONS

Hemolytic transfusion reactions may occur immediate or delayed. The latter type occurs in previously sensitized patients in whom no antibodies were detectable at the time of transfusion. However, following transfusion of incompatible donor red cells a secondary antibody response occurs and after about a week the antibody level is high enough to cause destruction of transfused red cells

* Supported in part by grants from the Dutch Cancer Society (Koningin Wilhelmina Fonds) and the Division for Health Research TNO.

which are still circulating. We might expect a decrease in frequency of hemolytic transfusion reactions as technological methods have been improved. However, data collected from an extensive series of patients in the Mayo Clinic from 1965 to 1980 (1) indicate no difference in the incidence (1:14,000 units transfused) of immediate reactions. On the other hand the delayed-type reactions were observed more frequently. The incidence increased from 1:11,600 transfusions in the period 1965–73 to 1:1,500 in 1978–80. This might reflect a greater awareness of the problem. On the other hand, it is possible that there is a real increase due to the fact that more patients have histories of previous blood transfusions.

Hemolytic transfusion reactions are potentially dangerous as they may be complicated by severe clinical problems, such as renal failure, disseminated intravascular coagulation and death. It has been reported that 17–40% of hemolytic transfusion reactions are fatal (1,2). The occurrence of a hemolytic transfusion reaction must therefore be considered to be a severe transfusion complication. The same conclusion may be drawn when we examine the etiology of transfusion associated fatality. In the period 1976–78 70 fatal reactions were reported to the Bureau of Biologics (3). There were 46 cases of hemolysis (two delayed) and this was found to be the major cause of transfusion fatality. Further investigations of these hemolytic reactions were performed to gain insight into ways of preventing these reactions and these revealed that incompatibility of the ABO-group was the major factor involved. As the determination of the ABO-group of patients is not difficult, and cross-match procedures should always detect incompatibilities, the question arises as to how these incompatibilities could occur. Human error is the major cause as errors have been detected at all levels in the procedure, ranging from faulty sample drawing to the administration of the wrong unit of blood. In only three of the 44 fatalities no error was detected.

It is obvious that error control should be the major objective in the prevention of acute reactions. This menas that all procedures, starting with the ordering from up to the eventual administration of the blood product should be designed to carry minimal risk of mistakes. Prevention of the delayed-type hemolytic transfusion reactions is more difficult as per definition no antibody is detectable at the time of cross-matching. It is thus essential to register any irregular antibody ever found in any patient, so that when this patient later on needs a blood transfusion and the antibody may no longer be detectable, blood without the corresponding antigen can be selected. Another approach would be the development of more sensitive cross-match procedures. It might then be possible to detect antibodies with very low titers.

FEBRILE NON-HEMOLYTIC REACTIONS

Febrile non-hemolytic transfusion reactions are much more frequent. It is estimated that these occur in 3% of all transfusions. Fever and chills develop within several hours of the start of the bloodtransfusion. The reaction results from destruction of granulocytes by anti-granulocyte antibodies (4) and may be prevented by using leukocyte-poor red cell preparations (5). However, the chance that a patient who has already experienced a febrile reaction has a similar reaction on the following transfusion is about 15% (6), so the use of these preparations is not mandatory after only one febrile transfusion reaction. If a patient has experienced two or three episodes, however, it is reasonable to prevent further reactions by administering leukocyte-poor preparations.

It is very important to realize that fever may also be the first sign of a hemolytic transfusion reaction (1). Thus, when fever develops the transfusion should always be stopped and hemolysis excluded.

ALLERGIC REACTIONS

Another frequently occurring reaction is the allergic transfusion reaction. Two forms do exist. The anaphylactic type is the most severe, but fortunately is rare. Patients may suffer from nausea, abdominal cramps, diarrhea and hypotension, but fever almost never develops. These reactions are mostly due to antibodies to IgA and occur in IgA-deficient patients (7). Transfusion should be stopped immediately and patients treated with epinephrine and other supportive measures. A diagnostic clue may be measurement of the IgA level in the recipient. These reactions may be prevented by the use of red cells, thoroughly washed for at least six times. When plasma is given to such a patient, it should be obtained from IgA negative donors.

The mild urticarial form is much more frequent. It is estimated to occur in 1 to 2% of transfusions, and is also thought to result from antibodies to plasma proteins. When this occurs the transfusion rate should be reduced or temporarily stopped and antihistamines should be given. When these reactions occur repeatedly prevention is possible by premedication with antihistamines.

PLATELET TRANSFUSION REACTIONS

Reactions after the administration of platelet transfusion may occur either due to the interaction of platelets and anti-platelet antibodies or to the presence of other components in the platelet suspension. The presence of a high titer of anti-A or anti-B antibodies in blood group O platelet preparations may lead to hemolysis when they are infused into an A or B group recipient (8). Febrile transfusion reactions following platelet transfusions may be caused by contaminating leukocytes and allergic reactions may be due to the presence of the plasma proteins. Immune-mediated destruction of the platelets are observed in the posttransfusion purpura syndrome and in alloimmunized patients.

Posttransfusion purpura is a delayed-type transfusion reaction. It is characterized by the onset of hemorrhages about a week after bloodtransfusion. On laboratory investigation severe thrombocytopenia is detected. Patients are usually female with a history of multiple pregnancies and/or bloodtransfusions. It is, however, curious that after bloodtransfusion the patients own platelets are evidently destroyed, and a mechanism for this phenomenon has been suggested by Shulman in 1961 (9). The postulated sequence of events is as follows: the patient lacks the platelet antigen P_1A_1, also known as Zw^a. When the patient receives a transfusion containing platelets, these platelets most probably will be P_1A_1 positive, as 98% of the population is P_1A_1 positive. In previously sensitized patients infusion of these platelets leads to development of anti-P_1A_1 antibodies as a secondary response. After about a week the antibody titer is high enough to cause destruction of the infused platelets and it is postulated that during this destructive process immune complexes of P_1A_1 antigen and anti-P_1A_1 antibodies are formed. These complexes then adhere to the recipients own platelets and thus lead to their destruction. This results in severe thrombocytopenia, which may last for two to six weeks. There is some evidence that plasma exchange may accelerate platelet recovery (10).

Another transfusion reaction involving platelets transfused, is platelet destruction in alloimmunized patients. Alloimmunization to platelets frequently occurs in patients who are repeatedly transfused. The frequency is estimated to be 50% although some authors mention even higher figures (11,12). The presence of allo-antibodies results in immediate destruction of transfused platelets and posttransfusion platelet increments are near zero. This means that further transfusions of random donor platelets are of no clinical value. To enable selection of donors based on HLA-typing, large pools of typed donors are needed and even then not all patients respond well to these transfusions. An alloimmunized patient thus runs an increased risk of hemorrhage and is a heavy burden on the supportive care unit. Prevention of alloimmunization would therefore be of great value.

Platelets carry both HLA-antigens and platelet specific antigens. Granulocytes and lymphocytes also carry HLA-antigens. This means that transfusion of granulocytes and lymphocytes may also lead to the development of anti-HLA antibodies, which cross-react with platelets. A first step in minimizing alloimmunization could be the elimination of leukocytes from red cell transfusions so that these are no longer immunogenic for the HLA-antigens (13).

The second point is whether we can modify the platelets themselves in order to delay alloimmunization. Such an approach could be based on the assumption that restriction of patient exposure to platelet antigens would decrease alloimmunization. Several options exist: one is to give platelets in case of bleeding only, the so-called therapeutic approach which reduces the number of transfusions compared to a prophylactic transfusion regimen. To date there are no data comparing these regimens in terms of development of both alloimmunization and hemorrhage protection. A study of this issue is in progress in our institute. A second option would be the use of special platelet preparations obtained from random single donors, from matched donors or lymphocytic-depleted suspensions.

When random single donor platelet preparations are used the recipient is exposed to a much smaller variety of platelet antigens per transfusion than in the usual 6–8 donor platelet suspensions. This could theoretically delay alloimmunization. We have performed a randomized trial on this subject (14). Patients with severe thrombocytopenia due to bone marrow depression were randomized to receive single donor or multiple donor platelets. We calculated the one hour posttransfusion recoveries, which are assumed to give a good indication of alloimmunization. The average platelet recoveries for the first and second transfusion in patients receiving single donor suspensions were the same. In contrast, there was a significant decrease in the posttransfusion platelet recoveries in the group of patients receiving multiple donor transfusions. We checked the patients for factors known to decrease recoveries such as fever, sepsis, splenomegaly and disseminated intravascular coagulation, but we could not detect any differences between the groups. Our interpretation of these data is that the decrease in recovery in the multiple donor group must be due to the development of antibodies. As recoveries remained constant in the single donor group, this suggests delayed alloimmunization by random single donor platelets. So far, these are the only data from a controlled clinical trial on random single donor platelet transfusions. As there are no data on patients receiving more than two transfusions, it is too early to recommend single donor platelets as a standard therapy with minimal alloimmunization.

Another technique in delaying alloimmunization could be the use of matched donors from the start of the transfusion therapy. This is not feasable in The Netherlands, as it is already very difficult to select a matched donor for a sensitized patient.

A different approach has been proposed by Eernisse's group in Leiden using platelet preparations which had been made as leukocyte poor as possible by extra centrifugation (15). This approach is based on the fact that lymphocytes are more immunogenic than platelets. Clinical results show that before 1974 when standard blood preparations were used, 90% of the patients became sensitized (26/28). However, after 1974, when both leukocyte-poor red cells and leykocyte-poor platelets were used the incidence of alloimmunization was much lower (16/68). It remains difficult to conclude that leukocyte-poor platelets per se will definitely delay alloimmunization. In this study historical controls were used. It is doubtful whether both study groups are comparable, as the use of leukocyte-poor red cells was introduced and cytotoxic treatment regimens have become more agressive, which might result in a decreased alloimmunization frequency. This assumption seems to be supported by the very high frequency of alloimmunization in the historical control group (90%) as compared to presently reported series in which the incidence of refractoriness is 40 to 50%. This would make the differences between the two approaches less pronounced.

In conclusion, approaches such as the use of single random donor platelets or leukocyte poor platelets are promising, but must be further investigated before they can be recommended as standard therapies.

GRANULOCYTE TRANSFUSION REACTIONS

Hemolysis may occur following granulocyte transfusion due to incompatible red cells contaminating the granulocyte suspension. In particular granulocyte suspensions prepared by centrifugation contain many red cells and red cell cross-matching should be performed. Allergic reactions may result from the presence of plasma. Granulocyte transfusions may lead to alloimmunization and anti-granulocyte antibodies may also influence the outcome of granulocyte transfusion. Fever frequently occurs after granulocyte transfusion. The incidence is influenced by variables such as collection method and rate of administration. Granulocytes prepared by centrifugation give a much lower incidence of fever and chills than leukocytes prepared by filtration. It is most probable that filtration prepared granulocytes are somewhat damaged by adhesion to the nylon filter. These reactions may be prevented by premedication of the recipient with antipyretics and/or corticosteroids. It is our policy to only premedicate patients that have already experienced febrile reactions. It has also been reported that rapid infusion of granulocytes results in more reactions than slow infusion (16).

Severe pulmonary complications may occur following granulocyte transfusion. Acute respiratory distress and pulmonary infiltrates may develop. It is generally assumed that these result from sequestration of transfused granulocytes in the pulmonary capillaries. There are several possible mechanisms for this phenomenon. One is that granulocytes migrate into an infected area of the lungs resulting in the appearance of a pulmonary infiltrate on the X-ray compatible with pneumonia (17). When leuko-agglutinins are present in the patient, clumping of granulocytes may occur and result in sequestration, and bilateral nodular infiltrates become visible on X-ray examination (18). It has also been postulated that there might be complement activation when circulating endotoxins are present in the recipient (19). This also results in granulocyte aggregation. A fourth mechanism is the direct infusion of aggregates present in the blood product. Aggregate-free granulocytes should be prepared and infusion of aggregates can be prevented by the use of standard blood filters (170 μ). The use of micro-aggregate filters should, of course, be omitted as they will retain the granulocytes. Corticosteroids are used for the treatment of these complications, and other supportive measures may be taken if necessary.

The majority of the reported cases of graft-versus-host reactions following bloodtransfusion have occurred following granulocyte transfusion in patients with severe immunodeficiency (20). It is an attack of immunocompetent lymphocytes on an immunocompromized host, and this reaction may occur after any transfusion containing viable lymphocytes. Indeed, these reactions have also been reported following red cell transfusion (21). The clinical findings which may arise suspicion of the presence of GVH are the development of a skin rash and diarrhea, and laboratory investigations may reveal liver function abnormalities. Confirmation of the presence of donor cells by genetic markers is diagnostic, although a skin biopsy may also be highly suggestive. GVH is a very serious form of transfusion reaction as it is very difficult to treat and the outcome is mostly fatal. Prevention may be achieved by irradiation of the blood product with 15–50 Gy. The question remains as to whether we should irradiate all blood products for all immunocompromized patients. Useful advice may be to irradiate all cell products for the most severely immunocompromized patients, for instance for patients with severe combined immunodeficiency and patients who undergo bone marrow transplantation, and to always irradiate granulocyte transfusions as these are usually given repeatedly and may contain very high amounts of lymphocytes.

CONCLUSIONS

It must be clear that the transfusion of blood or its components may result in a number of adverse immunologic reactions which may vary from mild discomfort to the death of the patient. It is very important to realize that most transfusion fatalities are due to human error and that they may be prevented by strict error control procedures both in the blood banks and in the hospital. The morbidity due to blood transfusion may be reduced by careful preparation of the product and also by the selection of the optimal blood product for each transfusion. Finally, it should be emphasized that the decision to administer blood or its components should only be taken when the expected benefits of the transfusion outweigh the possible risks.

REFERENCES

1. Taswell, H.F., Pineda, A.A., Moore, S.B. Hemolytic transfusion reactions: frequency and clinical and laboratory aspects. In: Bell, C.A. (ed.) A seminar on immune-mediated cell destruction. Am. Assoc. Blood Banks, 1981, pp. 71–92.

2. Baker, R.J., Moinichen, S.L., Nyhus, L.M. Transfusion reaction: a reappraisal of surgical incidence and significance. Ann. Surg. 1969;169:684–93.
3. Honig, C.L., Bove, J.R. Transfusion-associated fatalities: Review of bureau of biologic reports 1976–1978. Transfusion 1980;20:631–61.
4. Thulstrup, H. The influence of leukocyte and thrombocyte incompatibility on non-haemolytic transfusion reactions. Vox Sang 1971;21:233–50.
5. Brittingham, T.E., Chaplin, H. The antigenicity of normal and leukemic human leukocytes. Blood 1961;17:139–65.
6. Kevy, S.V., Schmidt, P.J., McGinniss, M.H., Workman, W.G. Febrile, nonhemolytic transfusion reactions and the limited role of leuko-agglutinins in their etiology. Transfusion 1962;2:27–16.
7. Vyas, G.N., Holmdahl, L., Perkins, H.A., Fudenberg, H.H. Serologic specification of human anti-IgA and its significance in transfusion. Blood 1969;34:573–81.
8. Mcleod, B.C., Sassetti, R.J., Weens, J.H., Vaithianathan, T. Haemolytic transfusion reaction due to ABO incompatible plasma in a platelet concentrate. Scand.J.Haematol. 1982;28:193–6.
9. Shulman, N.R., Aster, R.H., Leitner, A., Hiller, M.C. Immunoreactions involving platelets. V. Post-transfusion purpura due to a complement-fixing antibody against a genetically controlled platelet antigen. A proposed mechanism for thrombocytopenia and its relevance in autoimmunity. J. Clin. Invest. 1961;40:1597–1620.
10. Abramson, N., Eisenberg, P.D., Aster, R.H. Post-transfusion purpura: immunologic aspects and therapy. N. Engl. J. Med. 1974;291:1163–6.
11. Dutcher, J.P., Schiffer, C.A., Aisner, J., Wiernik, P.H. Long-term follow-up of patients with leukemia receiving platelet transfusions: Identification of a large group of patients who do not become alloimmunized. Blood 1981;58:1007–11.
12. Tejada, F., Bias, W.B., Santos, G.W., Zieve, P.D. Immunologic response of patients with acute leukemia to platelet transfusions. Blood 1973;42:405–12.
13. Diepenhorst, P., Engelfriet, C.P. Removal of leukocytes from whole blood and erythrocyte suspensions by filtration through cotton wool. V. Results after transfusion of 1,820 units of filtered erythrocytes. Vox Sang 1975;29:15–22.
14. Sintnicolaas, K., Vriesendorp, H.N., Sizoo, W. et. al. Delayed alloimmunization by random single donor platelet transfusions. A randomized study to compare single donor and multiple donor platelet transfusions in cancer patients with severe thrombocytopenia. Lancet 1981;1:750–4.
15. Eernisse, J.G., Brand, A. Prevention of platelet refractoriness due to HLA antibodies by administration of leukocyte-poor blood components. Exp. Hematol. 1981;9:77–83.
16. Djerassi, I., Kim, J.S., Suvansri, U., Ciesielka, W., Lohrke, J. Filtration leukopheresis: principles and techniques for

harvesting and transfusion of filtered granulocytes and monocytes. In: Goldman, J.H., Lowenthal, R.M. (eds.) Leukocytes: separation, collection and transfusion. Academic Press, New York, 1975, pp. 123–36.

17. Higby, D.J., Freeman, A., Henderson, E.S., Sinks, L., Cohen, E. Granulocyte transfusions in children using filter-collected cells. Cancer 1976;38:1407–13.
18. Ward, H.N. Pulmonary infiltrates associated with leukoagglutinin transfusion reactions. Ann. Intern. Med. 1970;73:689–94.
19. Higby, D.J., Burnett, D. Granulocyte transfusions: current status. Blood 1980;55:2–8.
20. Weiden, P.L., Zuckerman, N., Hansen, J.A. et. al. Fatal graft-versus-host disease in a patient with lymphoblastic leukemia following normal granulocyte transfusions. Blood 1981;57:328–32.
21. Dinsmore, R.E., Straus, D.J., Pollack, M.S. et. al. Fatal graft-versus-host disease following blood transfusion in Hodgkin's disease documented by HLA typing. Blood 1980;55: 831–4.

TRANSMITTABLE DISEASES AND BLOOD TRANSFUSION

H.W. Reesink

INTRODUCTION

Since the mid 1930s it has been recognized that human blood or plasma when administered to others may transmit serious bacterial or viral diseases. The use of normal human plasma as a stabilizer for vaccines was associated with massive epidemics of viral hepatitis. A yellow fever vaccine among American military personnel caused possibly over 40,000 cases of hepatitis in 1942.

Syphilis was often seen after direct transfusion of (uncooled) donor blood. Serious other bacterial infections in patients were also due to non-sterile transfusion equipment or anticoagulant solutions. Since then the risks of transmitting disease by blood have decreased in such a way that clinicians nowadays are often unaware of the possibility of transmitting infections to their patients by means of bloodtransfusion. This is especially true for those disease with a long incubation period.

The transfusion associated diseases are divided in three groups: viral, parasitic and bacterial.

TRANSMITTABLE VIRAL DISEASES

Viral diseases of major importance are hepatitis B, hepatitis non-A non-B (NANB), of occasional importance are cytomegalo virus (CMV) and Ebstein Barr virus (EBV) and of suspected importance are Lassa fever, Marburg and Ebola agents, slow viruses (Creutzfeldt Jacob, Kuru) and possibly the agent(s) causing the acquired immune deficiency syndrome (AIDS).

VIRAL HEPATITIS

Posttransfusion hepatitis (PTH) still is a major problem in bloodtransfusion. Since the discovery by Blumberg in the 1960's of the Australian antigen and the association of this antigen with hepatitis B virus (HBV) it became possible to develop specific tests to detect infectious donors, carrying the virus. In the 1970's serologic tests became available to detect hepatitis A virus (HAV) infections and it became clear that this virus did not play a role in PTH. It then became apparent that a considerable proportion of PTH still remained and that the PTH cases were neither caused by HBV, HAV, CMV or EBV. From epidemiologic and chimpanzee studies it was demonstrated that a transmittable agent or agents were responsible for these so-called NANB-PTH cases. Similar to HBV, an infectious carrier state for NANB agents exists in humans.

Usually the incubation time fo PTH-NANB is shorter (55d) than PTH-B (85d) although a large overlap between the two exists. In both disease 20–40% of the PTH-cases are icteric. An important percentage of the patients will develop chronic disease (chronic active hepatitis and cirrhosis). In PTH-B especially the non-icteric cases and in PTH-NANB the icteric cases with high liver enzyme levels (ALT) develop chronic disease. The acute disease of NANB is usually milder with lower ALT levels than in PTH-B. The significance of chronic NANB hepatitis is not fully understood at the moment. Although the majority of patients are classified as having chronic active hepatitis (CAH), they have in general, a clinically and histologically mild form of CAH. However, progression to cirrhosis has been documented in a few cases.

The incidence of PTH-B has decreased since the introduction of specific tests for HBsAg. In the USA the increased use of blood from unpaid donors instead of paid donors has decreased the number of cases of PTH dramatically. It has been shown that the use of blood and blood products from paid donors in the USA carries a 5–10 times higher risk of transmitting PTH-B as well as NANB. Prospective studies in the USA and Europe have shown that at the moment over 90% of all PTH cases are of the NANB type. The incidence in the USA of PTH-NANB is estimated to be between 5–8% (5–25 per 1000 units) in patients transfused with blood from unpaid donors and 25–50% (40–80 per 1000 units) in patients transfused with blood from paid donors (1,2).

In Europe very few prospective studies (3,4) have been carried out. They have shown that the incidence of PTH-NANB was comparable to the incidence found in the USA. When commercial blood products were transfused also a much higher frequency of PTH-NANB was found. In a prospective study in The Netherlands 13 observed cases of PTH-NANB were all non-icteric with no development to chronic hepatitis. Besides HBsAg for HBV, are there other markers associated with an increased incidence of PTH?

Anti-HBs positive blood from volunteers does not have an increased risk for PTH-B and NANB. There is a possible increased incidence for PTH-NANB when anti-HBs positive blood from paid donors is used (5). Anti-Hbc positive blood (without anti-HBs) is possibly associated with an increased risk for both PTH-B and NANB, although only limited data are available to substantiate this (6).

In many countries donors with a history of jaundice are rejected permanently because of possible increased risk for PTH, but no studies are available to justify this policy. In the United Kingdom and The Netherlands, countries which accept donors with a history of jaundice, serologic studies have shown that these donors have almost exclusively anit-HAV antibodies and also that they did not have an increased incidence of markers for HBV (7).

Since there is no specific test available to detect the NANB virus carriers, the question has arisen if serum alanine aminotransferase (ALT) levels could be used as a non-specific indicator of the NANB-carrier state among blood donors. Two prospective studies (8,9) in the USA, have shown that patients receiving blood from donors with an ALT value of less tan 2.25 times the standard deviation (SD) of the mean, had a significantly lower risk (6–9%) for PTH-NANB than patients transfused with blood from donors with an ALT value over 2.25 SD (29–45% risk for NANB-PTH). The PTH-NANB risk increases when the donor ALT values are higher and when more than one unit of blood with an elevated ALT is transfused. Although possibly 30% of PTH-NANB cases could be prevented by rejecting donors with elevated ALT's, it is important to emphasize that this is a predicted rather than a proved efficacy. Moreover 70% of the hepatitis cases will be uninfluenced by such testing and 70% of donors with elevated ALT's would be rejected without implication of hepatitis transmission.

Apart from the substantial loss of donors (3–5%) the costs per unit of blood would increase by 2–3 US dollars (10).

Freezing (and washing) of blood, advocated in some centres in the USA, has not shown to give a significant reduction of PTH, where it increases enormously in the costs.

Inactivation of the infectious agents responsible for PTH in donor blood is important. Human albumin solutions are "hepatitis free" since they are pasteurized for 10 hours at 60°C. Coagulation factor concentrates prepared from paid donor blood are known to cause PTH-NANB in a considerable proportion of the recipients. Some producers claim to have eliminated the hepatitis risk of these concentrates by heating or by the addition of gammaglobulin or beta-propriolacton.

HBV can be successfully eliminated by the addition of HBIG to blood products (11). An overdosage of 0.4 IU per ml anti-HBs proved to be sufficient to protect four chimpanzee's angainst hepatitis B, when injected with different products prepared from HBsAg positive plasma, while all the four control animals developed hepatitis B. It is uncertain, however, if gammaglobulin addition to blood (products) can give protection against NANB-PTH.

Since hepatitis B vaccins are available now, active immunization of recipients of blood (especially multiple transfused) may prevent PTH-B. The vaccination of donors against hepatitis B, although costly, will also safeguard the recipients against PTH-B. The elimination of PTH-NANB can only be reached when a specific test for the detection of the NANB-virus carriers has been developed.

CYTOMEGALO VIRUS (CMV)

It was noticed that after transfusion of many units of fresh blood (as in open heart surgery) recipients may develop 3–6 weeks later a mild illness associated with fever, non-icteric hepatitis, splenomegaly, neutropenia and the presence of atypical lymphocytes. The incidence of CMV infections after bloodtransfusion, is probably underestimated, because of the relative insensitivity of the complement fixation (CF)-technique and the fact that with this technique sera with anti-complement activity (most stored sera) cannot be tested. More sensitive indirect haemagglutination techniques show that in multiple transfused patients a "de novo" appearance of anti-CMV antibodies or a 4-fold rise in antibody titer can be demonstrated in 10–15% of open heart surgery patients. In patients developing PTH 30% could be diagnosed as CMV-infection. Therefore part of the earlier classified mild NANB-PTH cases were probably caused by CMV-infections (12).

The disease is self-limiting and only of importance in the immunocompromized host, e.g. renal transplant- and bone marrow transplant patients under immunosuppression and in newborn babies. In these patients it may cause severe (often lethal) illness (interstitial pneumonia, hepatitis, haemolytic anaemia). The incidence of CMV-antibodies in the normal population (in the CF-technique) is about 60%; 6–12% are actually excreting the virus in their urine and have infected leukocytes. The prevention of the disease is only indicated for immunosuppressed patients and newborns, i.e.: avoidence of fresh blood (products), removal of leukocytes from blood or donor selection (for exchange transfusions in newborns). Hyperimmune CMV immunoglobulin has been shown to protect immunocompromized patients against CMV-infections (13).

EBSTEIN-BARR VIRUS (EBV)

The disease, which is self-limiting, may develop as PTH in susceptable recipients receiving multiple bloodtransfusions. EBV-infections may only play a role in immunosuppressed individuals. At present these infections are not a significant problem in bloodtransfusion, because 30–70% of the normal population have antibodies to EBV. The disease must be discriminated from PTH-B, NANB and CMV.

However, it should be stressed that the virus has a co-carcinogenic potential (Burkit lymphoma), in which the role of transfusion transmitted infection is unknown.

VIRAL DISEASE OF SUSPECTED IMPORTANCE (14,15)

Some degree of viraemia is present in most human viral infections but are not of interest in bloodtransfusion. A few serious viral infections, although not associated with bloodtransfusion, should be considered because of future possible epidemics and importation from the areas in question.

LASSA FEVER

Lassa fever is caused by an arena-virus infection in West-Africa, identified in 1969. Viraemia may occur (2–3 weeks) in clinical cases and persistent infections were demonstrated in people born in the endemic area (West-Africa). The virus may be transmitted by blood contact during the period of viraemia.

MARBURG AND EBOLA AGENTS

Marburg and Ebola agents are rhabdo viruses; clinical infections are found in Central Africa but have also been seen in laboratory associated outbreaks in Europe (1967). The mortality rate is high (20–40%). The natural host is unknown. A prolonged viraemia of 2–3 months has been observed in secondary parenterally exposed humans.

ARBO VIRUSES

Arbo viruses are transmitted by one vertebrate host to another by hematophagus arthropods. Over 300 different viruses are known of which 80 have been isolated from humans as disease source. The best knwon disease caused by this group of viruses is Colorado tick fever (CTF) occurring exclusively in the Western USA and Canada. Viraemia may vary from several weeks to several months. No cases until now of CTF are reported to be associated with bloodtransfusions.

SLOW VIRUSES

Although there is no evidence that diseases associated with slow virus infections (Creutzfeldt-Jacob (CJD), Kuru) are transmitted by bloodtransfusion, CJD may be transmitted by corneal transplant procedures in humans and apes.

ACQUIRED IMMUNE DEFICIENCY SYNDROME (AIDS)

Since 1979 a new syndrome has been identified the so-called Acquired Immune Deficiency Syndrome (AIDS). Patients involved have a cellular immune deficiency, together with an opportunistic infection (mainly pneumocystis carinii) and/or Kaposi sarcoma. Like hepatitis B virus transmission, homosexuals and bisexuals with multiple different sexual contacts are at risk. Further intravenous drug abusers, Haitians reciding in the USA and haemophilia patients receiving Factor VIII concentrates were attacked.

Between june 1981 and september 1982 593 cases of AIDS were reported. Death occurred in 243 (41%). There is practically no survival two years after diagnosis. Every half year the number of cases doubled, indicating that an infectious agent (viral?) is responsible for transmission of the disease. It may be possible that blood and blood products are means to transmit the disease. Especially products derived from pools of many donors (coagulation factor concentrates) are of major concern. So far no infectious agent could be identified and primate transmission studies have failed to transmit the disease (16).

PARASITIC DISEASES (14,15)

The most important parasitic diseases transmitted by blood are malaria and Chagas disease and will be discussed. Others (African trypanosomiasis, Filariasis, Kala-Azar, Toxoplasmosis, Babesiosis) are rarely reported to be transmitted by blood and will not be discussed.

Malaria

It is estimated that more than 100 million people in the world are infected with malaria parasites and that about one million patients per year die from the disease. In Europe and the USA the disease is only imported by infected persons coming from endemic areas (see WHO-map). In the literature more than 2000 cases of transfusion associated cases of malaria are described, the majority after 1960. The risk per million units of blood is estimated to be 0.8 in the USA, 0.2 in the UK and 4.0 in France (15).

Since 1971 an alarming increase of posttransfusion malaria cases due to P. falciparum was observed in the USA and in France. This is of importance because practically all reported cases of death from PT-malaria were caused by P. falciparum. P. malariae and P. vivax are now much less found in PT-malaria and P. ovale is very rarely found in transfusion accidents. A problem is that the diagnosis of PT-malaria often takes a very long time (3–4 weeks of the average). The virulence of the parasite is proportional to the immune deficiency of the patient. All transfusions requiring fresh blood seem to increase the danger, but blood stored for at least ten days at 4°C is not associated with transmission of PT-malaria. Prevention of PT-malaria is mainly achieved by fixing time limits for rejection of donors coming from malaria endemic areas. The Council of Europe (15) recommends the following time limits:

- six months after return if the subject is asymptomatic and has not taken a course of chemoprophylaxis;
- three years in all other cases, including immigrants.

AREAS OF RISK FOR MALARIA TRANSMISSION, DECEMBER 1976

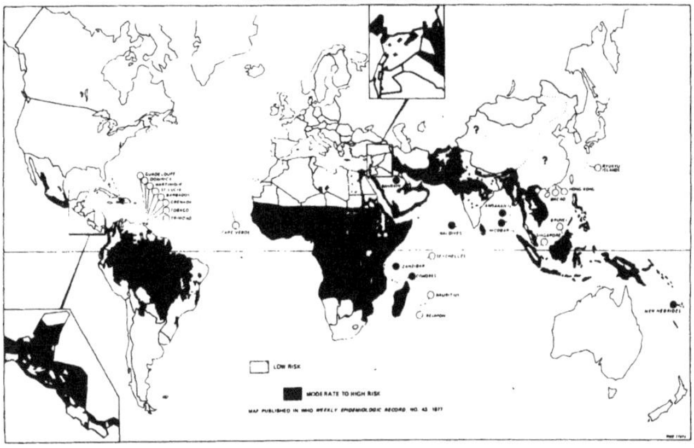

With these measure the risk for PT-malaria and especially P. falciparum infections, will be significantly reduced.

Chagas disease

This trypanosomiasis, caused by Trypanosoma cruzii, is only found in the north of South America. It is estimated that there are about 7 million carriers of the parasite. The disease may be fatal in children and in adults it may lead to chronic disease affecting the heart and the nervous system, 5–9% of carriers are found in these areas. CF-antibody tests may detect 95% of the chronic and 50% of the acute forms. The disease is associated with transfusion of fresh blood; blood after ten days storage is regared to be safe. Also addition of a 1:4000 dilution of gentian violet to blood destroys the parasite within 24 hours.

BACTERIAL DISEASES (14,15,17)

Bacterial disease transmitted by blood may be caused by a bacteriemia in the donor, i.e. syphilis or by a transitory bacteriemia (e.g. after tooth extraction) mainly with Gram positive bacteria. Case reports have described the transmission by blood of borreliae, brucellosis, salmonellosis and Yersinia enterocolica.

Syphilis

Before 1946 several hundred cases of posttransfusion syphilis (PTS) were reported. However, since that time almost no new cases of PTS have been observed. In 1979 in the USA it was therefore questioned whether serological testing for syphilis in blood donors ought to be continued. The main reason for the decreased incidence of PTS are probably refrigeration of blood and the use of antibiotics in transfused patients.

One may question if the screening of syphilis antibodies and exclusion of the positive donors really contributes to the decrease of PTS.

Arguments against screening are:

- In spirochetaemia there is a long (4–9 weeks) sero-negative phase.
- Serum positivity does not always mean spirochetaemia.
- High cost to benefit ratio.
- Exclusion and loss of donors because of the existence of so-called biological false positives and haemagglution assay (TPHA) positives (serological scars).

Arguments in favour of testing are:

- The increasing use of fresh blood (products like platelets).
- The prevention of the disease (in donors).

The Council of Europe (15) recommends, however, maintenance of systematic screening for syphilis in donors.

Another suggestion could be to test all patients for syphilis antibodies 4–6 weeks after transfusion. This is, however, not feasible.

Other bacterial infections

More important and dangerous bacterial infections may be caused by contamination of blood equipment, punctures in the closed system, improper storage of blood (products) (especially in the hospital wards) and the danger of re-issuing blood for different patients. Although older studies have shown that 1–3% of the blood collected in plastic bags and up to 20% of platelet concentrates stored at room temperature are contaminated with bacteria, transfusion reactions resulting from these contaminations are rare.

85% of the transfusion accidents in patients are due to Gram negative bacteriae, whereas these bacteriae are responsible for only 13% of all the cases of contaminated blood. The most common Gram negative bacteriae found in transfusion accidents are: achromobacters (58%), pseudomonas (21%), Escherichia freundii (11%), coli forms (8%) and E. coli (2%).

Over 50% of these transfusion reactions are fatal, causing severe (warm) shock and disseminated intravascular coagulation, mainly due to endotoxins from the bacilli. The most important measures to prevent bacterial contamination are: maintenance and control of refrigeration (also in the hospitals), no opening of the closed system before transfusion, inspection of the blood unit for an abnormal colour or haemolysis, and limitation of storage periods for platelet concentrates kept at room temperature.

REFERENCES

1. Vyas, G.N., Cohen, S.N., Schmid, R. Viral Hepatitis. Franklin Institute Press, Philadelphia, 1978, pp. 371–81, 383–96, 405–14.
2. Robinson, W.S. The enigma of non-A/non-B hepatitis. J. Inf. Diseases 1982;145:387–95.
3. Sugg, U., Erhardt, S., Lissner, R., Schneider, W. Incidence of posttransfusion hepatitis type non-A/non-B in the Fed. Rep. of Germany. Proc. 19th Congr. ISH/17th Congr. ISBT, Budapest, august 1982.
4. Tremolada, F., Chiapetta, F., Noventa, F., Valfre, C., Ongaro, G., Realdi, G. Prospective study of posttransfusion hepatitis in cardiac surgery patients receiving only blood or also blood products. Vox Sang 1983;44:25–30.
5. Gerety, R.J. Non-A/non-B Hepatitis. Academic Press, New York, London, San Francisco, 1981, pp. 63–4.
6. Rakela, J., Mosley, J.W., Aach, R.D. et al. Gastroenterology, 1980;78:1318.
7. Aach, R.D., Alter, H.J., Barker, L.F. et al. Should donors with a history of jaundice still be rejected? Int. Forum Vox Sang 1981;41:110–27.
8. Aach, R.D., Szmuness, W., Mosley, J.W. et al. Serum alanine aminotransferase of donors in relation to the risk of non-A/non-B hepatitis in recipients. The transfusion-transmitted viruses study. New Eng. J. Med. 1981;304:989–94.
9. Alter, H.J., Purcell, R.H., Holland, P.V., Alling, D.W., Koziol, D.E. Donor transaminase and recipient hepatitis. Impact on blood transfusion services. JAMA 1981;246:630–4.
10. Aach, R.D., Bayer, W.L., Gerety, R.J. et al. Based on your analysis of the benefits and costs of routine donorscreening for ALT-GPT to reduce the incidence of posttransfusion non-A/non-B hepatitis in your blood service region, what action would you recommend on this matter? Int. Forum Vox Sang 1983; 44:48–64.
11. Brummelhuis, H.G.J., Over, J., Duivis-Vorst, C.C. et al. Contributions to the optimal use of human blood. Vox Sang (in press).
12. Alter, H.J., Purcell, R.H., Feinstone, S.M., Tegtmeier, G.E. non-A/ non-B hepatitis: its relationship to cytomegalovirus to chronic hepatitis and to direct and indirect test methods. In: Szmuness, W., Alter, H.J., Maynard, J.E. (eds.) Viral Hepatitis. The Franklin Institute Press, New York, London, San Francisco, 1981, pp. 279–94.
13. Condie, R.M., O'Reilly, R.J. Prophylaxis of CMV-infection in bone marrow transplant recipients by hyperimmune CMV gammaglobulin. Develop. Biol. Standard 1982;52:501–13.
14. Greenwalt, T.J., Jamieson, G.A. Transmissible disease and blood transfusion. Grune & Stratton, New York, San Francisco, London, 1975.

15. Council of Europe: Assessment of the risks of transmitting infectious diseases by the international transfer of blood, its components and derivatives. 1980 Co-ordinated Blood Transfusion Research Programme.
16. CDC Update on acquired immune deficiency syndrome (AIDS)-United States. MMWR 1982;31:507–14.
17. Mollison, P.L. Blood transfusion in clinical medicine. 6th ed., Blackwell Scientific Publ. 1979, pp. 647–54.

PLATELET TRANSFUSION: QUALITY CONTROL

Ch.A. Schiffer

Platelets for transfusion are prepared either as a byproduct of whole blood donation from multiple donors as platelet concentrates (PC) or using mechanical blood cell separators which prepare large numbers of units form single donors. The available blood cell processors consistently produce platelets of good functional and morphologic quality which are usually administered shortly after collection (1,2,3,4). The major issues of "quality control" relate primarily to proper maintenance and utilization of the machine so as to ensure consistent platelet yields and donor safety. Because all of the available blood cell separators are "open systems", single donor platelets cannot be stored for more than 24 hours prior to transfusion and long-term storage is therefore not currently a major issue. When such platelet preparations have to be transported long distances under varying conditions of temperature and agitation or when greater than 12 hour storage is contemplated, it is best that the platelets be collected in a large, 2000 ml bag to provide increased surface area for gas exchange (5).

In most blood centres, however, the great majority of platelets administered are prepared as platelet concentrates (PC). It is the collection and storage of these preparations which provide the greatest difficulties and which will be discussed in this commentary. Numerous reports have documented that under proper circumstances PC can be stored for up to three days at ambient (22–24°C) temperature with maintenance of posttranfusion viability and hemostatic function (6,7,8,9). More recently, the development of thinner plastic bags with increased permeability to oxygen and carbon dioxide have been developed which now permit storage with satisfactory maintenance of viability for up to five days (10,11). It should be noted, however, that even in these carefully conducted studies in research laboratories, there is often considerable variability in the results achieved posttransfusion with stored platelets. Although there is a paucity of published data, it is likely that this variability is even greater in large blood centres (12,13). This is particularly true because platelet collection, preparation and storage is now frequently done on a large, "assembly line" scale which may no longer command the specialized attention it received when platelet transfusion represented innovative technology.

Table I. Factors influencing platelets (PC) during storage.

1. Collection techniques – particularly second centrifugation, method of resuspension.
2. Temperature.
3. Platelet concentration (plasma volume).
4. Agitation; separation of bags.
5. Type and size of container.
6. Transport.
7. Degree of WBC contamination.

A large number of factors can potentially adversely affect platelet concentrates during storage. In addition to the factors listed in Table I, there may be individual features in particular donors which are obviously difficult to assess. In this regard, investigators in platelet research laboratories not infrequently note unexplainable differences in platelet function from apparently "normal individuals". A number of the "simple" steps involved in platelet separation from whole blood can also significantly affect platelets during storage. The centrifugation speeds and times used to prepare platelet-rich plasma (PRP) and subsequently PC vary considerably amongst different blood centres (14). Although it is likely that very little platelet injury occurs during PRP formation because the platelets are "sedimented" against the RBC cushion, there is also variation in the policy with regard to how close to the red blood cells PRP collection is done. Although platelet yields probably increase as the RBC layer is approached, with most centrifugation speeds the WBC yield in the bags is also increased (15). Increased WBC or possibly RBC contamination may contribute to enhanced overall metabolism in the PC and more rapid fall in pH during storage (16). In addition, denser, larger platelets may be collected in greater numbers as the RBC are approached. Although it may be theoretically desirable to collect these possibly younger platelets (17), a recent study has demonstrated that there is little difference in posttransfusion survival between PRP enriched with the slightly larger platelets harvested near the RBC layer and PRP collected at a higher level in the bag (18). Furthermore, there is a suggestion that these more metabolically active platelets may contribute disproportionately to lactate production during storage thereby accelerating the fall in pH (15). Further studies are necessary to confirm these findings and to provide more precise guidelines.

It is likely, however, that it is the second centrifugation to prepare PC which is more critical in terms of platelet injury. Slichter and Harker have demonstrated that "softer, slower" centrifugations are preferable to "harder, shorter" spins in terms of maintenance of platelet viability (2,19). Many blood banks have to prepare large numbers of PC over short periods of time and therefore compromise with these centrifugation suggestions in order to process PC more rapidly. Time constraints also probably influence the means in which PC are resuspended in many centres. Ideally, the PC should be left at rest on a table for one to two hours prior to being placed on a shaker for storage, thereby allowing aggregates which may have formed during centrifugation to break up. Lastly, the majority of whole blood collections are done in mobile units distant from the blood centre and the site of component production. Delays in transport, temperature changes, etc. can all potentially influence the quality of platelets produced.

Temperatures in blood banks frequently vary widely according to season and the racks upon which the platelets are suspended in many cases do not permit adequate separation of the bags with free circulation of air. Increased availability of room temperature incubators with to-and-fro agitators have helped to standardize what was often an enormously disparate approach to platelet storage. In general, these requirements for agitation, physical separation of the bags, and avoidance of excessively high concentrations of platelets in the PC by using adequate plasma volumes are all designed to help guarantee adequate oxygen delivery to the platelets (15,20). Decreases in plasma O_2 with resulting anaerobic metabolism is associated with accumulation of lactate, fall in pH and loss of viability and clinical effectiveness. There is also debate about which method of agitation of PC is preferable so as to minimize injury to platelets caused by repeated contact with the walls of the bag (15,20). Currently, horizontal to and fro agitation at a rate of approximately 70/min is probably preferable (19,20). Because donor platelet counts are not (and need not) be routinely measured, the plasma volume should be at least 50 to 60 ml to help minimize the likelihood of excessive concentration of platelets. Even so, in donors with higher counts, many units will have greater than 1.6×10^6 platelets/μl, a concentration which is often associated with rapid falls in pH and loss of viability even after short duration of storage (6,9,15,19,20). Because most transfusions consist of 4–10 units of PC, however, the inclusion of occasional units such as this should not substantially affect the overall results of most transfusions.

The metabolic and functional changes occurring during platelet storage have been extensively studied and are summarized in Table II. Morphologically, as the pH of stored PC falls, there is progressive swelling of the platelets with dendrite formation (21). Although best detected by electron microscopy, these changes can also be well-characterized by careful phase microscopic evaluation or by cell sizing studies. These morphologic changes are also associated with decreased cell density probably related to transmembrane leakage of solute (22,23). Even afger relatively brief (24 hours) storage at room temperature, there is a well-described decrease in response to aggregating agents and decreased release

Table II. Structural and functional changes during storage.

1. Progressive swelling, decreased density (21,22,23).
2. Decrease in aggregation response and release reaction (6,24, 27).
3. Loss (? alteration) of membrane glycoproteins (28,29).
4. Decreased adenine nucleotides particularly in metabolic pool (30,31).
5. Leakage (? release) of beta-TG, PF-4, LDH (32).
6. Minimal loss of cholesterol, phospholipids (33).
7. Minimal changes in contractile proteins (34).

of serotonin and nucleotides after appropriate stimuli (6,15,24). Recently, however, it has been demonstrated that a normal aggregation response can occur when two aggregating agents, such as collagen and ADP are added simultaneously. This is perhaps analogous to what may occur in vivo (25,26). The mechanism for the decreased responsiveness is unclear although some studies have suggested loss of receptors for thrombin (27). This may in turn be related to alterations in membrane glycoproteins which occur progressively during storage. In addition, some studies have demonstrated "energy pool" depletion of adenine nucleotides, particularly in the metabolically active pool. The addition of adenine to the plasma (i.e. as in CPD-A1 anticoagulant) does not adversely affect platelets during storage (9,35).

In spite of these seemingly profound in vitro changes, PC which have maintained an adequate pH during storage (probably greater than 6.0 and certainly greater than 6.1–6.2) can have almost normal recovery and survival posttransfusion. In addition there are data to suggest that many of these apparent defects are correctable posttransfusion because transfused platelets collected from thrombocytopenic recipients can aggregate normally in vitro (6). Perhaps more critically, in terms of selecting a suitable quality control assay, it has been difficult to demonstrate a precise correlation between either simple or complex in vitro measurements and posttransfusion behaviour. This is particularly true of all of the functional assays. With respect to simpler measurements, there is a clearcut association at the extremes between the pH of PC and posttransfusion viability. PC in which the pH has fallen to 6.0 or below are nonviable and will not circulate after transfusion. This fall in pH is related to the large variety of conditions which in individual bags can produce poor oxygenation. Conversely, bags in which the pH has risen (greater than 7.5) are also likely to contain largely non-viable and often aggregated platelets, The most common cause of this phenomenon, particularly with the new thinner bags, is rapid efflux of CO_2 often in association with an initially low bag platelet count (10). What is unclear, however, is whether more subtle damage occurs due to the extensive metabolic processes which result in pH's in the 6.1 to 6.2 level. Although it has been shown that under some circumstances such platelets can circulate normally, it is not known how universal a phenomenon this is. Therefore, pH provides only a very rough guide to posttransfusion behaviour. There is a suggestion that protection against falls in pH by the addition of buffering devices can help protect platelets against irrevocable damage despite the fact that active metabolic processes continue (23,26).

Ordinarily, platelets circulate in a thin discoid shape. Platelets which are stored at 4°C or collected in EDTA anticoagulant rapidly become spherical in shape due to dissolution of microtubules and have a marked decrease in posttransfusion survival (24). Other studies have domonstrated that platelets which have become spherical during storage also have decreased recovery and survival (20,21). Kunicki et al. have described a morphologic grading system which roughly correlates different degrees of worsening platelet morphology with poorer posttransfusion viability (37). More recently, Holme and Murphy have described methodology using a platelet aggregometer to quantitate the relative number of discoid and spherical platelets in a given platelet preparation (23). They have also shown a correlation between preservation of discoid morphology and posttransfusion circulation. These techniques can be particularly helpful in the evaluation of more experimental platelet preparations and we have utilized such morphologic assessments in our evaluation of different techniques of platelet cryopreservation (38). However, except for examples in which there is gross distortion of platelet morphology, it is difficult to utilize morphologic techniques in more routine blood banks for quality control purposes.

Lastly, it should be mentioned that blood banks must remain aware of the rare (38,39) but real (40,41) problem of bacterial contamination of PC ocurring at the time of collection with further proliferation during storage. Obviously careful attention must be paid to sterility at the time of collection and processing. Clinicians should be cognizant that patients who have an unusually severe reaction following infusion of stored platelet should have the transfusion discontinued. Bag and blood cultures should be done and antibiotics begun if clinically appropriate.

Perhaps because of all of these inherent difficulties, regulatory agencies in the United States have imposed rather minimal criteria for platelet quality control assessment. Thus, serial platelet counts and pH have to be measured in a few units of platelets per month after storage for 72 hours. Notably absent from the guidelines is mention of clinical follow-up of results of platelet transfusion. The intent of platelet transfusion is to provide prophylaxis against and treatment of hemorrhage in thrombocytopenic patients. There is a linear relationship between the platelet count and the bleeding time which is currently the only *in vivo* test of hemostatic function (42). Bleeding times are difficult to perform and uncomfortable for the patient, particularly when done repeatedly, and do not demonstrate a good relationship with the onset of hemorrhage in severely thrombocytopenic patients. Freqeunt bleeding times therefore cannot be recommended as part of routine follow-up of the results of platelet transfusion.

Measurement of posttransfusion increments is obviously a potentially simpler means of assessing the likelihood of hemostatic effectiveness. It is now well accepted that monitoring of platelet counts immediately and 18 to 24 hours after transfusion is the most reliable means of determining the need for and the results of attempts to provide histocompatible platelets for alloimmunized recipients (43). Few if any blood banks, however, do this in a systematic fashion in an attempt to obtain similar information about the posttransfusion behaviour of stored platelets provided by their blood centre (44). Because it is the practice in most centres to utilize prophylactic transfusions for relatively stable, nonalloimmunized patients, it should be possible in most large centres to identify suitable patients for evaluation of the quality of both fresh and stored platelets. Ideally, a standardized corrected increment should be utilized. The formula utilized in our institution (1,43) is a corrected increment (CI) where:

$$CI = \frac{\text{Absolute increment x body surface } (m^2)}{\text{number of platelets transfused x } 10^{1}}$$

Thus if an absolute increment of 40,000 was achieved in a 2 m^2 recipient following the infusion of $4x10^{11}$ platelets, the CI = 40,000x2/4 = 20,000. Normally, a CI of approximately 18–22,000 should occur utilizing fresh platelets in stable nonalloimmunized patients without splenomegaly. If consistently lower increments are obtained then blood banks should carefully restudy collection and storage procedures and modify them as appropriate. Assessments of this sort should become a routine part of platelet transfusion practice. Obviously collection of this data depends upon collaboration between practicing physicians and the blood banks and it is important that close working relationships be established. Platelet transfusion is an expensive therapeutic modality with a number of adverse side effects and closer collaboration is clearly in the interest of improved patient care. Parenthetically, it should also be noted that blood banks do not charge different prices for stored as compared to fresh platelets. It is also the practice of many blood centres to transfuse "older" platelets first in the interest of inventory control so as to minimize platelet wastage. This practice may have particular relevance as the use of "five-day" platelet bags expands. There is presently very little information about the efficacy of platelet stored for five days in these bags except for the reports from the initial research laboratories. Although the overall results were satisfactory, there was considerable variability in the results from patient-to-patient. It remains to be seen what the results will be in the general blood bank setting. Because there are relatively few circumstances in which blood banks should find it necessary to keep platelets for five days, it may well be that the very important benefit of these newer platelet bags will be to help guarantee a more reliable platelet product after storage for 48 to 72 hours. If so, some of the variables listed in Table I may have a less profound deleterious influence on platelet viability after storage. It is important that blood centres utilizing these bags monitor pH, bag counts, possible WBC counts and posttranfusion results at greater frequency than thy have done in the past (and with considerably greater frequency than required by current US regulations) so as to more rapidly determine the most effective fashion in which these new platelet bags can be utilized.

REFERENCES

1. Daly, P.A., Schiffer, C.A., Aisner, J., Wiernik, P.H. A comparison of platelets prepared by the Haemonetics Model 30 and multiunit bag plateletpheresis. Transfusion 1978;19:778–81.
2. Slichter, S.J. Efficacy of platelets collected by semi-continuous flow centrifugation (Haemonetics Model 30). Brit. J. Haem. 1978;38:131–40.
3. Katz, A.J., Genco, P.V., Blumberg, N. et al. Platelet collection and transfusion using the Fenwal CS-3000 Cell Separator. Transfusion 1980;21:560–3.
4. Kalmin, N.D., Grindon, A.J. Pheresis with the IBM 2997. Transfusion 1980;21:325–9.
5. Katz, A., Houx, J., Ewald, L. Storage of platelets prepared by discontinuous flow centrifugation. Transfusion 1978;18: 220–33.
6. Murphy, S., Gardner, F.H. Platelet storage at 22°C; Metabolic, morphologic, and functional studies. J. Clin. Invest. 1971;50:370–7.
7. Slichter, S.J., Harker, L.A. Preparation and storage of platelet concentrates. Brit. J. Haem. 1976;34:403–19.
8. Pilip, D.J., Aster, R.H. Relative hemostatic effectiveness of human platelets stored at 4° and 22°C. J. Lab. Clin. Med. 1978;91:618–24.
9. Scott, E.P., Slichter, S.J. Viability and function of platelet concentrates stored in CPD-adenine (CPDA-1). Transfusion 1979;20:489–503.
10. Murphy, S., Kahn, R.A., Holme, S. et al. Improved storage of platelets for transfusion in a new container. Blood 1982;60: 194–200.
11. Blajchman, M.A., Kelton, J.G., Senyi, A.F. et al. The maintenance of hemostatic function, survival, platelet membrane glycoproteins and pH of human platelet concentrates stored for 5 days in new polyvinyl chloride blood bags. Blood 1981; 58:178 (abstract).

12. Lazarus, H.M., Herzig, R.H., Warm, S.E., Fishman, D.J. Transfusion experience with platelet concentrate stored for 24 to 72 hours at 22°C. Importance of storage time. Transfusion 1982;22:39–43.
13. Patel, I.P., Ambinder, E., Holland, J.F., Aledort, L.M. In vitro and in vivo comparison of single-donor platelets and multiple-donor pooled platelets transfusions in leukemic patients. Transfusion 1978;18:116–9.
14. Kahn, R.A., Cossette, I., Friedman, L.I. Optimum centrifugation conditions for the preparation of platelet and plasma products. Transfusion 1976;16:162–5.
15. Moroff, G., Friedman, A., Robkin-Kline, L. Factors influencing changes in pH during storage of platelet concentrates at 20–24°C. Vox Sang. 1982;42:33–45.
16. Beutler, E., Kuhl, W. Platelet glycolysis in platelet storage. Transfusion 1980;20:97–100.
17. Corash, L., Shafter, B., Perlow, M. Heterogeneity of human whole blood platelet subpopulations. I. Relationship between buoyant density, cell volume, and ultrastructure. Blood 1977; 49:71.
18. Mezzano, D., Kwang, K., Aster, R.H. Characteristics of total platelet populations and of platelets isolated in platelet-rich plasma. Transfusion 1982;22:197–202.
19. Slichter, S.J., Harker, L.A. Preparation and storage of platelet concentrates. Brit. J. Haem. 1976;34:395–402.
20. Holme, S., Vaidja, K., Murphy, S. Platelet storage at 22°C: Effect of type of agitation on morphology, viability, and function in vitro. Blood 1978;52:425–35.
21. Holme, S., Murphy, S. Quantitative measurements of platelet shape by light transmission studies; application to storage of platelets for transfusion. J. Lab. Clin. Med. 1978;92: 53–64.
22. Bolin, R.B., Cheney, B.A., Simpliciano, O.A., Smith, D.J. Buoyant density of platelets stored at room temperature as platelet concentrates. J. Lab. Clin. Med. 1981;98:342–51.
23. Holme, S., Murphy, S. Platelet storage for transfusion at 22°C: Interrelationship of platelet density and size, medium pH, and viability after in vivo infusion. J. Lab. Clin. Med. 1982 (in press).
24. Slichter, S.J. In vitro measurements of platelet concentrates stored at 4 and 22°C: Correlation with posttransfusion platelet viability and function. Vox Sang. 1981;40:72–86.
25. Moroff, G., Chang, C.H. Aggregation response of human platelets stored at 22°C as platelet-rich plasma. Transfusion 1979;19:704–18.
26. DiMinno, G., Silver, M., Murphy, S. Stored human platelets retain full aggregation potential in response to pairs of aggregating agents. Blood 1982;59:563–8.
27. White G.C., Workman, E.F., Lundblad, R.L. The effect of ambient storage on platelet membrane structure and response to thrombin. Transfusion 1979;19:411–9.

28. Jamieson, G.A., Ordinas, A. Surface components of platelets and their changes during storage. Vox Sang. 1981;40:18–21.
29. George, J.N. Platelet membrane glycoproteins: alteration during storage of human platelet concentrates. Thromb. Res. 1976;8:719–24.
30. Rao, A.K., Niewiarowski, S., Murphy, S.: Acquired granular pool defect in stored platelets. Blood 1981;57:203–8.
31. Kotelba-Witkowska, B., Holmsen, H., Murer, E. Storage of human platelets: Effects on metabolicaly active ATP and on release reaction. Br. J. Hematol. 1972;22:429.
32. Synder, E.L., Hezzey, A., Katz, A.J., Bock, J. Occurrence of the release reaction during preparation and storage of platelet concentrates. Vox Sang. 1981;41:172–7.
33. Hamid, M.A., Kunicki, T.J., Aster, R.H. Lipid composition of freshly prepared and stored platelet concentrates. Blood 1980;55:124–30.
34. Lucas, R.C., Lawrence, J., Stracher, A. On the preservation of contractile proteins during storage of human platelets. Blood 1981;57:1005–10.
35. Wong, S.C., Rock, G. The effect of adenine on platelet storage. Transfusion 1982;22:283–7.
36. Kotelba-Witkowska, B., Harmening-Pittiglio, D.M., Schiffer, C.A. Storage of platelet concentrates using ion exchange resin charged with dibasic phosphate. Blood 1981;58:537–43.
37. Kunicki, T.J., Tuccelli, M., Becker, G.A., Aster, R.H. A study of variables affecting the quality of platelets stored at "room temperature". Transfusion 1975;15:414.
38. Kotelba-Witkowska, B., Schiffer, C.A. Cryopreservation of platelet concentrates using glycerol-glucose. Transfusion 1982;22:121-4.
39. Silver, H., Sonnenwirth, A.C., Beisser, L.D. Bacteriologic study of platelet concentrates prepared and stored without refrigeration. Transfusion 1970;10:315–6.
40. Buchholz, D.H., Young, V.M., Friedman, N.R. et al. Bacterial proliferation in platelet products stored at room temperature. Transfusion induced Enterobacter sepsis. N. Eng. J. Med. 1971;285–429.
41. Blajchman, M.A., Thornley, J.H., Richardson, H. et al. Platelet transfusion-induced Serratia Marcescens sepsis due to vacuum tube contamination. Transfusion 1979;19:39–44.
42. Harker, L.A., Slichter, S.J. The bleeding time as a screening test for the evaluation of platelet function. N. Eng. J. Med. 1972;287:155.
43. Daly, P.A., Schiffer, C.A., Aisner, J., Wiernik, P.H. Platelet transfusion therapy: One-hour posttransfusion increments are valuable in predicting the need for HLA-matched preparations. JAMA 1980;243:435–8.
44. Schiffer, C.A. International Forum: What are the parameters to be controlled in platelet concentrates in order that they may be offered to the medical profession as a standardized product with specific properties? Vox Sang. 1981;40:122–4.

CLINICAL EFFICACY AND SAFETY OF FACTOR VIII CONCENTRATE

J-P. Allain

The clinical efficacy of Factor VIII therapeutic preparations has never been formally established since no controlled trial has ever been done comparing a preparation containing biological Factor VIII activity and a control. However, years of replacement therapy with whole blood, plasma, cyroprecipitate and concentrate have provided evidence for their efficacy. The clinical evaluation of these products is always difficult in hemophiliacs due to the rarity of open hemorrhages leaving the clinician with criteria such as pain, joint movements or joint circumferences to estimate efficacy.

A few years ago one study attempted to demonstrate the relationship between Factor VIII:C levels in the patients' circulation and clinical outcome on joint and muscle hemorrhages (1). The relationship seemed to be an exponential where 20% of circulating VIII:C correspond to 80% clinical success and 40% of circulating VIII:C to 97% success rate. Similarly an exponential relationship was demonstrated between the dose of Factor VIII injected calculated in U/kg body weight and the clinical outcome. These results suggested that the in vitro measurement of VIII:C in therapeutic products was a reliable indication for its clinical efficacy.

The number of Factor VIII preparations available to the clinician is quite large and as many as 20 different products made with different purification techniques are available in Europe. Since these techniques might affect the in vitro and in vivo behaviour of Factor VIII each preparation should be carefully studied both in vitro and in vivo.

In vitro, Factor VIII:C measurement in the products can be done either by one or two-stage assay provided the appropriate standard is used. For testing cryoprecipitate, a plasma pool or a cryoprecipitate can be used as standard calibrated against the WHO plasma standard. For testing concentrates, only a concentrate should be used as reference after calibration against the WHO concentrate standard.

In vivo, both biological and clinical studies are to be done. The measurement of VIII:C in sequential plasma samples from severe hemophilia A patients treated with a suitable dose of Factor VIII aims at evaluating Factor VIII recovery and Factor VIII half-life. Several technical precautions are required to obtain valid results and the items to be considered are listed in Table I.

Table I.

Patient selection	(bleeding or not bleeding)
Dose injected	($\geq$ 20 U/kg)
Sampling	
Measurement of Factor VIII:C	
Calculation of recovery and half-life	

There is a certain variation of VIII:C behaviour from patient to patient and it might increase when they are bleeding. However, when a hemorrhage is limited to a small capacity joint, no significant difference can be demonstrated. Sampling is important in its schedule and its actual collection. Early samples, post-infusion (15, 30, 60 min) allow the pick up the maximum Factor VIII plasma level to be used in the calculation of recovery; late samples (4, 12, 24, 36 hours) are required to calculate the Factor VIII half-life. Blood samples are drawn and processed so that the aliquots of plasma can be stored below -25°C within 60 minutes. Once all samples from one infusion are collected, they should be tested in one session with the same calibrated plasma standard.

Calculation of in vivo recovery is made in two ways, which are in good agreement in most cases. One is based on the assumption that one unit of VIII:C injected per kg body weight provides 0.02 U/ml VIII:C in the circulation. The second relies on the estimation of plasma volume with various methods of calculation. The number of units of VIII:C infused divided by the plasma volume in ml gives a theoretical value in units for the peak of circulating VIII:C. Both methods provide an expected VIII:C plasma level. The actual recovery expressed in percentage is therefore:

$$\frac{\text{measured VIII:C plasma level x 100}}{\text{expected VIII:C plasma level}}$$

Factor VIII half-life can be obtained by various mathematical calculations. In any case it should be done on the basis of VIII:C values from at least 4 plasma samples collected at 4 hour post-infusion and later.

Such studies have been done in our laboratory for a large number of Factor VIII preparations available in Europe. Table II shows a classification of these products according to potency and specific activity (ration U VIII:C/mg of proteins).

Several brands of commercial products in each category have been tested in vivo in patients with minor hemorrhages as defined above. Doses varying from 15 to 30 U/kg were infused in at least

Table II. Proposed definition of Factor VIII containing therapeutic products.

Name	VIII:C potency U/ml	Range of specific activity U/mg
Cryoprecipitate	2-10	0.1-0.4
Intermediate purity concentrate	20	0.5-0.9
High purity concentrate		
a	20	1 -2
b	20	> 2

three different patients for each product. As shown in Table III, no significatn difference appears for in vivo recovery which is always close to the expected 100%. Factor VIII half-life is slightly longer with cryoprecipitate but no significant differences exist among the various types of concentrates.

In our experience, all preparations were clinically efficacious. Possible differences in efficacy can only be demonstrated by proper double blind trial which has not yet been performed.

To day, where increasing consumption of Factor VIII preparations and spreading of long-term prophylaxis is generally accepted, the safety of therapeutic products draws an increasing attention. The problem is not so much immediate side effects (pyrogen reaction, allergy, etc.) which have decreased with the use of concentrates, but rather the long-term side effects. They are related to either contaminating proteins present in the Factor VIII preparations or to the presence of infective agents such as viruses related to hepatitis.

Table III. In vivo recovery and half-life of Factor VIII:C in patients treated with Factor VIII preparations.

Product	Number of brands studied	In vivo recovery %	VIII:C half-life mean (range)
Cryo	2	100	12 (10-15)
Intermediate purity	5	97–107	9.8 (8-14)
High purity a	5	91-102	10.4 (7-14)
High purity b	2	96-101	9.2 (8-11)

Table IV shows the main contaminating proteins found in Factor VIII preparations. These five proteins are present in various amounts in all products and account for 70-99% of the total proteins. Fibrinogen, fibronectin and albumin are essentially harmless to the recipient; immunoglobulins G or M are the almost exclusive source of side effects.

Table IV. Main contaminating proteins in Factor VIII preparations (% of total proteins).

Product	Fibrinogen	Fibronectin	Albumin	IgG	IgM	Total
Cryo	60.4	22	6	7.2	2.4	98
Intermediate purity concentrate						
1	49	21	14.6	10.8	2	97
2	48.8	34	12.2	10.3	2	95
3	43	6.1	23.7	11	5.5	89
4	47.4	16.3	13.3	10.1	1.2	88
High purity concentrate a						
1	28	33	0.3	30	4.2	96
2	36	41.4	0.7	5.7	1.3	85
3	70	17.7	2.2	8.9	1.7	97
High purity concentrate b						
1	80	1.8	3.2	8.6	7.7	101
2	25.3	18.1	4	23.2	7.7	78

IgG represents 6-30% of the total protein content and IgM 1-8%. The consequences of repeated infusions of these products appear at two levels. IgG coming from a large number of donors contain all possible Gm and Inv antigenic determinants. Some of them are not born by the recipient, but originate from immunization against foreign determinants. The infused IgG and IgM have a large number of specificities, some of them being possibly harmful to the recipient. Blood group A and B allo-agglutinins are an example, when infused to a group A, B or AB recipient.

Hemophilic populations have been studied in terms of anti Gm and anti Inv antibodies and 40-50% of those who are multitransfused carry such antibodies (5,10). When receiving IgG containing blood products IgG-anti IgG complexes are formed. The pathogenicity of these complexes is not demonstrated but some authors have related renal disease and repeated hematuria to circulating immune complexes in hemophiliacs (12). However, many other antigens can be involved in these circulating immune complexes. Their incidence in hemophiliacs have been studied by several

Table V.

Author \ Method	% of positives PEG	CIq	Raji cell binding	Protein A
McVerry 1977	62	94		
Kazatchkine 1978	62	16		
Poskitt 1981			48	
Verroust 1981		16	22	
Hilgartner 1982			50	90

authors with various techniques. Some of these results are indicated in Table V.

The role of passively infused immunoglobulins is also clinically relevant. Blood group allo-agglutinins have been shown by many authors to be responsible for hemolysis. However, it is recognized that only large doses of Factor VIII injected over a period of at least three days provoke a progressive decrease of hematocrit and hemoglobin possibly misleading the clinician for a hemorrhage. Factor VIII preparations, although made of large pools of plasma, vary largely in their anti A and anti B allo-agglutinin titers. In our centre, anti A titers in freeze dried cyroprecipitate vary from 1:2 tot 1:62 and in Factor VIII concentrate from 1:4 to 1:256. In average, anti B titers are lower than anti A by one dilution. When injected in A, B or AB recipients, these products induce a progressive hemolysis with positive direct Coombs test and positive elution test. Various means have been used to prevent hemolysis:

Table VI. Anti A and anti B antibody titers in Factor VIII concentrates.

Plasma pool	Specific acitivity (U/mg)	Nb of lots tested	Titers anti A	anti B
Unselected	0.5-0.9	10	16-128	8-32
	1 -2	3	4- 32	4-16
	2	3	32	16-32
Selected group A	0.5-0.9	2	2	2- 4
	1 -2	10	0- 2	1-16
	2	1	2	8

neutralisation with group specific substances, selection of low titer lots of concentrate, none of them being satisfactory. The only efficient method is to make pools of plasmas of the same blood group. This particular is feasible for blood group A and results of allo-agglutinin titers measured in concentrates made out of unselected and selected plasma pools are presented in Table VI.

It is to be emphasized that moderate hemolysis rapidly overcome by increased red cell production, does not seem to be pathogenic and its prevention has relatively rare indications.

The second large chapter concerning the safety of Factor VIII concentrate is the transmission of hepatitis. The magnitude of the problem is given by the high incidence of permanent or occasional high levels of transaminases in hemophiliacs as shown in Table VII.

Table VII. Incidence of liver dysfunction in hemophiliacs.

	ALT levels (% of total)		
Author	normal	elevated occasional	permanent
Levine 1976	49	23	28
Hasiba 1977	11	40	44
Parquet 1981*	75	19	6

* This population of 88 hemophiliacs is treated on demand only with large pool cryoprecipitate from voluntary blood donors.

The frequency of abnormal transaminases relates in part to the frequency of treatment episodes and to the origin of the plasma. It is essentially related to hepatitis B and non-A non-B. Most authors agree on an 80% incidence of HBV markers whatever the type of product used. However, the use of third generation tests for the detection of HBsAg in donors has significantly reduced the risk for a similar number of infusions (Parquet 1981). The main risk is now considered to be non-A non-B hepatitis, which seems to be responsible for most clinical and chronic hepatitis. Little can be done to prevent non-A non-B hepatitis since no reliable screening test is available at the moment. Several attempts to reduce or eliminate the risk of transmitting viral hepatitis are made. In France vaccination against hepatitis B is done systematically in new diagnosed hemophiliacs. Specific antibodies develop in most of them after three injections at one month interval. Another approach is the inactivation of both B and non-A non-B viruses by physical or chemical means. One concentrate treated by heat has recently been presented. The yield of Factor VIII:C seems to be less than 15%, but the in vivo recovery and half-life is not significantly affected. The efficacy of this type of process has to be clinically demonstrated in appropriately selected populations with special regard to non-A non-B.

In conclusion the Factor VIII concentrates available to the patient all seem to be equally efficacious. Important improvements are still required in terms of safety mainly by removal of immunoglobulins and of hepatitis viruses.

REFERENCES

1. Allain, J-P. Dose requirements for replacement therapy in hemophilia A. Thromb. Haemost. 1979;42:825–31.
2. Allain, J-P., Verroust, F., Soulier, J.P. In vitro and in vivo characterization of Factor VIII preparations. Vox Sang. 1980;38:68–80.
3. Hasiba, U., Spero, J.A., Lewis, J.H. Chronic liver dysfunction in multitransfused hemophiliacs. Transfusion 1977;17: 490–9.
4. Kazatchkine, M.D., Sultan, Y., Burton-Kee, E.J., Mowbray, J.F. Circulating immune complexes containing anti-VIII antibodies in multi-transfused patients with hemophilia A. Clin. Exp. Immunol. 1980;39:315–20.
5. Kernoff, P.B.A., Bowell, P.J. Gm types and antibodies in multi-transfused haemophiliacs. Brit. J. Haematol. 1973;24: 443–50.
6. Levine, P.H., MacVerry, B.A., Attock, B., Dormandy, K.M. Health of intensively treated hemophiliacs with speical reference to abnormal liver chemistries and splenomegaly. Blood 1977;50:1–9.
7. Mannucci, P.M., Capitanio, A., Del Ninno, E., Colombo, M., Pareti, F., Ruggeri, Z.M. Asymptomatic liver disease in hemophiliacs. J. Clin. Pathol. 1975;28:620–4.
8. Parquet-Gernez, A., Boulanger-Fasquelle, P., Maniez-Montreuil, M., Goudemand, M. Etude des marqueurs sanguins biologiques des hépatites virales chez 157 hémophiles. Reve. Franç. Immunohématol. 1981;24:463–82.
9. Poskitt, T.R., Poskitt, P.K.F., Bean, C.A., Arkel, Y.S. Immune complexes in hemophilia. Am. J. Haematol. 1981;11: 147–52.
10. Verroust, F., Adam, C., Kourilsky, O., Allain, J.-P., Verroust, P. Circulating immune complexes and complement levels in hemophilic children. J. Clin. Lab. Immunol. 1981;6:127–30.
11. McVerry, B.A., Voke, J., Mohammed, I., Dormandy, K.M. Immune complexes and abnormal liver function in haemophilia. J. Clin. Pathol. 30:1142–6.
12. White, G.C., Blatt, P.M., McMillan, C.W. et al. Medical complications of haemophilia. South Med. J. 1980;73:155–63.

THE USE OF INDIUM-LABELED GRANULOCYTES TO HELP ASSESS THE CLINICAL EFFICACY OF GRANULOCYTE TRANSFUSIONS

M. Clay, J.F. McCullough

INTRODUCTION

A major problem associated with the use of granulocyte transfusion therapy has been the lack of a method to evaluate their clinical efficacy. In vivo kinetic studies of granulocytes radiolabeled in vitro have been performed in human subjects with either ^{32}DFP or ^{51}Cr (1,2,3,4,5). ^{32}DFP is a relatively specific label for granulocytes that has been widely used until recently when it became commercially unavailable. Chromium-51 labeling studies have given differing results due to the indiscriminate labeling of leukocytes, platelets, and red blood cells. Although external body counting is possible with ^{51}Cr, the dose limitations with the use of this radioisotope make external organ imaging impractical.

Indium-111-oxine is an efficient label for leukocytes (6,7). Indium-111 has a t 1/2 of 67 hours and emits gamma photons in high abundance which are nearly ideal for external imaging. Because of this, the use of indium-labeled leukocytes is increasing in popularity for detection of inflammation and abscess. Since indium-oxine labels leukocytes, red blood cells, and platelets in varying degrees, its usefulness for kinetic and organ localization studies of granulocyte transfusions depends on the preparation of a pure granulocyte suspension.

Indium-labeled granulocytes (^{111}In-granulocytes) can be used to study the effect of different variables which may be important in the success of granulocyte transfusions. The effect of leukocyte antibodies on the fate in vivo of granulocytes is not known. Antibodies to non-red cell antigens found on leukocytes can be detected by many techniques, but the comparative value of these different techniques for detection of immune destruction of granulocytes in different clinical situations is not known (8). In granulocyte transfusion, early studies showed that when patients had leukoagglutinating or lymphocytotoxic antibodies, imcompatible granulocytes had a decreased intravascular recovery and failed to localize at sites of infection (9,10,11). However, the clinical effectiveness

* Supported in part by Contract #N01-HB-6-2972 and Grant #5-R01-HL-26568-02 from the National Heart, Lung and Blood Institute and a research grant from the American National Red Cross.

of granulocyte transfusions was apparently not related to HLA compatibility (12), and leukocyte antibody testing did not protect the recipient from a transfusion reaction (13,14).

With the development of techniques for collection and transfusion of granulocytes, the changes that occur in granulocytes during storage have become more important. Although much has been learned about granulocyte function in vitro, little is known about the in vivo effectiveness of stored granulocytes. When granulocytes are stored at 1-6°C for 24 hours, there is a reduction in the percent which circulate following transfusion (15,16), and approximately 75% reduction in the number which migrate into a skin abrasion (16); while storage at 20-24°C provides better maintenance of in vitro chemotaxis (17,18).

In this report, we describe the preparation and labeling of an essentially pure granulocyte suspension to study the intravascular recovery, survival time, and extravascular localization of ^{111}In-granulocytes. In order to determine the effect of different leukocyte antibodies on the fate in vivo of granulocytes, we have studied the intravascular kinetics and extravascular localization of ^{111}In-granulocytes in pateints with different kinds of leukocyte antibodies, and have combined the use of ^{111}In and a skin window blister technique to study the fate in vivo of stored granulocytes.

MATERIALS AND METHODS

Preparation and labeling of granulocytes

A relatively pure granulocyte suspension was prepared with the use of a discontinuous Ficoll-Hypaque gradient as previously described (19). Granulocytes were processed from 125 ml ACD whole blood obtained by phlebotomy or from granulocyte concentrates which were collected from normal subjects by leukaphereses using continuous flow centrifugation or intermittent flow centrifugation with hydroxyethyl starch. The subjects were not premedicated with steroids. The suspension contained a range of 1-3x10^8 granulocytes with less than 1% mononuclear leukocytes and less than 5% red blood cells. No hypotonic lysis of red blood cells was used.

Indium-111-oxine was prepared (19) by mixing ^{111}In chloride with 50 ml of 8-hydroxyquinoline (oxine) (1 mg/ml ethanol) and 0.2 ml 0.3 M sodium acetate buffer (pH 5.5). After extraction with chloroform, the extract was evaporated to dryness and the residue taken up in 50 μl of ethanol and diluted with 0.3 ml of saline.

The granulocyte suspension was labeled with an average of 200 μ Ci of ^{111}In-oxine by incubation in a sterile vial at room temperature for 20 min with occasional gentle mixing. The labeled granulocytes were then withdrawn through a needle containing a filter and injected through an ordinary needle into the recipient. The small amount of labeled cell suspension remaining in the vial was used to determine labeling efficiency and the number of cells injected.

Intravascular recovery and t 1/2 determination

Blood samples were obtained from the recipient at approximately 10 min, 1, 2, 3, 4, 5, and 6 hours after injection, and the granulocyte-associated radioactivity was determined. Because the injected radioactivity is either firmly bound to granulocytes or free in the supernatant, the cell-associated radioactivity can be determined by subtracting the plasma value from the whole blood activity. The determination of the percentage of recovery of granulocytes and their t 1/2 was based on total cell-associated activity injected and the recipient's blood volume as previously described (19).

Body distribution of ^{111}In-granulocytes

Extravascular localization of the injected granulocytes was determined by whole body imaging. Body scans were performed occasionally at 4 hours and always at 24 hours after injection, using either a whole body scanner or a scintillation camera.

Effect of leukocyte antibodies

On the morning of the indium study, blood was obtained from the recipients and from normal donors. A cross-match between recipients' serum and the donors' granulocytes or lymphocytes was done that day. The granulocyte microagglutination assay (GA) and the granulocyte cytotoxic assay were performed as previously reported (8,20). Lymphocytotoxicity (LC) testing was done using standard techniques (21). Details of this study have been previously published (20).

Briefly, patients were grouped based on the kind of antibody present, the presence of neutropenia, and the presence of infection. The mean value for recovery and t 1/2 for each group was determined. Each group of patients with antibodies was compared with a group of patients matched for the presence or absence of neutropenia and infection but with no antibodies. Differences between groups were evaluated using a t test with 2-4 degrees of freedom. Differences were considered significant if $p < 0.05$, but very large differences in means would be necessary to achieve statistical significance in groups with small numbers of patients.

In order to evaluate the accuracy of the indium scan, the patients' subsequent clinical courses were monitored. X-ray and laboratory data and findings at surgery or autopsy were accumulated and a final decision was made whether, in retrospect, each patient had a localized infection at the time of the indium study. Each indium scan was then classified as a true-positive (if the patient was infected and granulocytes localized at the site of infection), true negative (if the patient was not infected and granulocytes failed to localize anywhere other than the liver and spleen), false-positive (if granulocytes localized at a site that did not give evidence of infection), or false-negative (if granulocytes failed to localize at a known site of infection).

Storage of granulocytes

Granulocytes for storage studies were obtained and prepared as mentioned above and previously published (22). The granulocytes that were studied without storage were resuspended in 5 ml of saline and immediately labeled with ^{111}In-oxine. For storage studies, the isolated granulocytes were resuspended in 12 ml of thawed CPD fresh frozen plasma and stored in a 150 ml transfer bag (Fenwal) at 1-6°C or 20-24°C for 8 hours or 24 hours. After storage, the granulocyte plasma suspension was centrifuged, washed once with saline to remove residual plasma, and then resuspended in 5 ml of saline for labeling.

Skin window assay of in vivo chemotaxis

Evaluation of in vivo chemotaxis of ^{111}In-granulocytes was performed using a modified skin window technique that we have previously described in detail (22). Three 8 mm diameter blisters were formed on the volar surface of the forearm by gentle heat and suction. The blister roof was removed aseptically and a leucite chamber was secured in place over each lesion. One ml of autologous serum in each chamber served as the chemoattractant for subsequent intravenously injected Indium-labeled autologous granulocytes. The chambers were left in place for 24 hours after which the serum was removed. The number of ^{111}In-granulocytes in the chamber was evaluated in two ways (22). The percent of injected ^{111}In-granulocytes recovered in the chambers (percent migration) was determined to give an indication of the overall ability of injected granulocytes to migrate into the chambers. The ability of those cells which did circulate to migrate into the chambers was evaluated by calculating a Migration Index (MI) based on the average number of ^{111}In-granulocytes in the circulation during the 24 hours the skin chambers were in place.

For subjects in whom granulocytes were not stored, the skin windows were created immediately after the granulocyte donation. Subjects who received stored granulocytes went about their normal activities after leukapheresis, then returned the following morning (or after 8 hours) for placement of the skin windows and injection of the stored ^{111}In-granulocytes.

These studies were approved by the University of Minnesota Committee on the Use of Human Subjects in Research. All participants gave informed consent. All donors of granulocytes met the criteria of the American Association of Blood Banks for ordinary blood donation and were HBs antigen negative.

RESULTS

Intravascular recovery and survival

Studies of the intravascular kinetics of ^{111}In-granulocytes were performed in 10 normal subjects (Table I). An average of 11×10^7 granulocytes were labeled with approximately 200 microcuries of ^{111}In. Approximately 89% of the injected radioactivity was associated with the granulocytes and 11% remained free in the supernatant solution. The intravascular recovery of ^{111}In-granulocytes was 30 ± 5.9% and the half-life was 5.0 ± 1.6 hours. The average value of 30% is the observed maximum recovery and is not based on projections to zero time.

Table I. Kinetics of ^{111}In-granulocytes in ten normal subjects*

Number of granulocytes injected ($\times 10^7$)	11 ± 6
Indium-111 radioactivity (microcuries)	100 ± 80
Labeling of granulocytes (percent)	89 ± 4
Intravascular recovery (percent)	30 ± 5.9
Intravascular half-life (hours)	5.0 ± 1.6

*From (22) with permission.

The half-life of the indium-labeled granulocytes in the circulation was determined by plotting the decrease in cell-associated radioactivity in the circulation, as shown in Figure 1. In 8 of the 10 subjects, the maximum level of radioactivity in the circulation did not occur until an hour to 2 hours after injection. The half-life

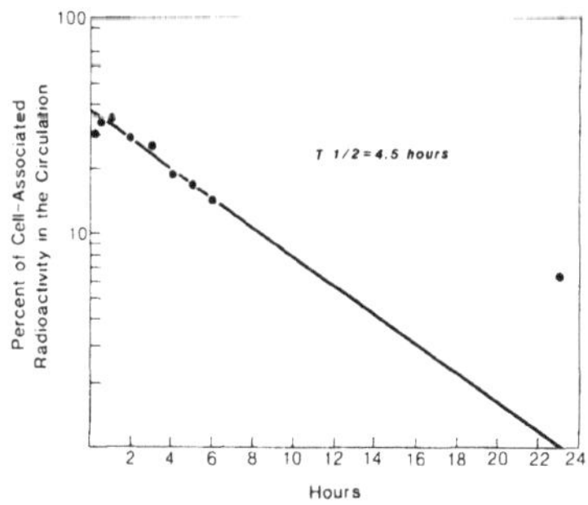

Figure 1. Intravascular disappearance of ^{111}In-granulocytes in an individual normal subject (from (22) with permission).

was determined over the most linear portion of the plot. The intravascular cell-associated radioactivity plateaued between 6 and 24 hours, so that the radioactivity present at 24 hours was consistently higher than expected.

Body distribution

In 10 normal subjects, body scans were performed at approximately 4 and 24 hours after transfusion of autologous ^{111}In-granulocytes to determine their organ localization (19). There was accumulation of radioactivity mainly in the liver and spleen, and no evidence of uptake in the lungs at 24 hours. However, when camera images were obtained in the first 1 to 2 hours after transfusion, some lung activity was evident. In 4 of the 10 patients, there was visable uptake of radioactivity in the bone marrow of the pelvis and spine after 24 hours.

In one study of body distribution, a series of images were obtained immediately following injection of ^{111}In-granulocytes in a normal subject (23). The camera was positioned posteriorly to include the liver, spleen, and lungs; images were then obtained every 30 seconds for the first 90 minutes. The first image (Figure 2A) was obtained during the first 30 seconds after injection and shows a bolus of radioactivity in the subclavian vein and some in the heart and lungs. In the next 30second image (Figure 2B), there is a high degree of activity in the lungs and some activity in the spleen. Figure 2C, which was obtained 3 minutes after injection, shows activity in both the spleen and liver. The lung activity decreased rapidly, so that by 90 minutes (Figure 2D) most of the activity was in the liver and spleen.

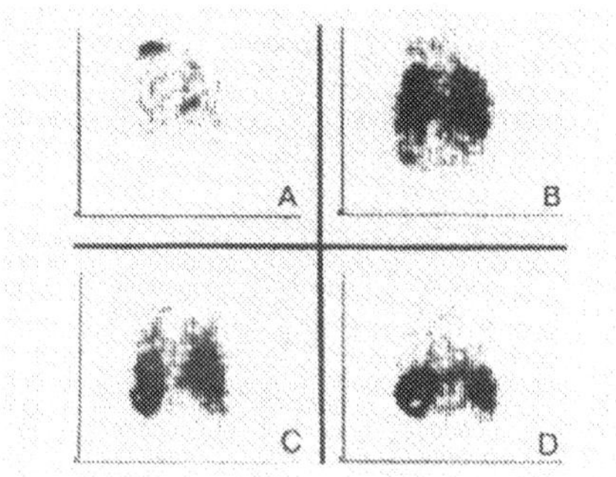

Figure 2. Posterior views of camera images obtained over the chest area at 30 second intervals following injection of ^{111}In-granulocytes. A. 0-30 seconds after injection; B. 30-60 seconds after injection; C. 3 minutes after injection; and D. 90 minutes after injection. (From (22) with permission).

Abscess localization

Satisfactory in vivo function of ^{111}In-granulocytes has been previously established at our institution by studies of 406 patients in which localization at confirmed sites of inflammation or abscess occurred in 140 of 155 patients (24). This represented a test sensitivity of $\sim$ 90%. There were 19 cases in which localization of activity on ^{111}In-leukocyte scans was not definitely correlated with acute inflammation and 15 cases in which autologous ^{111}In-granulocytes failed to localize at known sites of infection. The calculated specificity was thus $\sim$ 93%, yielding an overall diagnostic accuracy of approximately 91%.

Effect of leukocyte antibodies

This previously reported study (20) involved a total of 50 patients; 25 adult and 25 pediatric who received 58 injections of ^{111}In-granulocytes. Patients were neutropenic (< 1000 PMNs/μl) during 36 of the 58 studies. In 25 studies, the granulocytes injected were compatible by the three antibody methods (GA, GC, LC), and in 32 studies, the granulocytes were incompatible in one or more assays. Body scans were obtained in all studies and intravascular recovery and t 1/2 of the labeled granulocytes were determined in 31 studies. Follow-up evaluation indicated 31 sites of infection in 25 studies and no localized infection in 33 studies.

In order to establish a base for comparison, patients who received granulocytes compatible in the GA, GC and LC crossmatches will be considered first. Kinetics data were obtained in 15 patients. In the 6 non-neutropenic patients, the average intravascular recovery was 30.0% in the absence of infection and 31.7% in the presence of infection with an average t 1/2 of 8.8 hours and 4.8 hours, respectively (Table II). These values are similar to the 30% recovery and 5.0-hour half-life we previously reported in normal subjects receiving autologous granulocytes (19). The three infected patients had decubitus ulcers, infected central venous pressure line, and numerous large boils. Neutropenic patients with no antibodies had significantly reduced recoveries when compared with similar non-neutropenic patients with no antibodies (Table II): uninfected, 15.6% versus 30.0%; $p < 0.01$ and infected, 11.0% versus 31.7%, $p < 0.01$). There was no statistically significant difference among the t 1/2 for these groups of patients with no antibodies.

Sixteen patients with leukocyte antibodies were studied, and the results are compared with the values for the 15 patients without antibody (Table II). Four patients received granulocytes incompatible by GA. In the 3 non-neutropenic uninfected patients, the intravascular recovery (10.5%) and t 1/2 (2.0 hour) were significantly less ($p < 0.01$) than in similar patients without antibodies (30%, 8.8 hours). In one of these patients, the GA antibody had anti-NB1 specificity, and NB1-positive donor granulocytes had a significantly reduced ($p < 0.05$) recovery (14.4%) and a t 1/2

Table 2. Intravascular recovery and half-life of ^{111}In-granulocytes in 16 studies when leukocyte antibodies were present and 15 studies when no antibodies were detected by granulocyte agglutination (GA), granulocytoxicity (GC), or lymphocytotoxicity.

Cross-match result* GA	GC	LC	Neutropenic	Infection present	Number of studies	Percent of recovery	Hours half-life
-	-	-	No	No	3	30.0	8.8
-	-	-	No	Yes	3	31.7	4.8
-	-	-	Yes	No	4	15.6	4.4
-	-	-	Yes	Yes	5	11.0	6.1
+	-	-	No	No	3	10.5	2.0
+	-	-	Yes	No	1	6.4	1.1
-	+	-	No	No	1	27.8	-
-	+	-	Yes	No	2	18.7	2.9
-	+	-	Yes	Yes	3	17.9	4.5
-	-	+	Yes	Yes	1	5.1	2.3
+	-	+	Yes	Yes	1	4.0	1.2
-	+	+	Yes	No	4	12.1	5.5

* A minus indicates no reaction between recipient's serum and donor cells, and thus, indicates a compatible transfusion, while a plus indicates incompatibility.

of 2.4 hours ($p < 0.05$). The intravascular recovery and t 1/2 in the one neutropenic patient with GA antibody was reduced but not significantly different from similar patients without antibodies (6.4% versus 15.6%; $p > 0.05$). Studies in 6 patients with GC antibodies also showed differences between neutropenic and non-neutropenic patients, but none of the recovery or t 1/2 values was different from similar patients with no antibodies (non-neutropenic 27.8% versus 30.0%; neutropenic uninfected 18.7% versus 15.6%; and infected 14.1% versus 11.0%). One neutropenic infected patient received granulocytes imcompatible by LC. Although the recovery was less than those in patients without antibodies (5.1% versus 11%), the differences were not significant ($p > 0.05$). The one patient with both GA and LC antibodies also had a low recovery that was not statistically significant (4% versus 11%; $p > 0.05$). Four neutropenic uninfected patients who had both GC and LC antibodies had a recovery and t 1/2 (12.3% and 5.5 hours) similar to those seen in neutropenic uninfected patients with no antibodies (15.6% and 4.4 hours).

Probably more important than survival in the intravascular space is the granulocyte's ability to migrate to a site of infection. Of the 58 indium studies reported here, 25 were done in patients with clinically proven infection. Twenty-three of these were detected by the indium scan and considered true-positives, but two were missed and thus were false-negatives (Table III). Both of these patients had GA antibodies; one in combination with GC and one in combination with LC. The GA antibody that was present with the GC antibody had anti NA1 specificity. This patient had osteomyelitis (confirmed by a bone scan) of the pelvis and an AK amputation stump. NA1-positive ^{111}In-granulocytes did not localize at those sites. In the second patient with a false-negative scan, an LC antibody was present with the GA antibody. Granulocytes failed to localize at an area of clinically apparent submandibular cellulitis.

None of the 4 patients with GA antibodies alone had localized infections, so that all of the scans in these patients were true-negatives. GC antibodies were present in 10 studies. Five of these patients had known sites of infection and demonstrated localization of ^{111}In-granulocytes at these sites (Table III). One patient had pneumonia demonstrable by chest X-ray, one had oral and anal ulcers and pseudomembranous colitis (Figure 3), one had an inflammed thermal burn, one had a lung abscess, and one was undergoing rejection of a transplanted kidney. There were no false-negative studies in patients who received GC incompatible granulocytes.

Six patients had LC antibody and two of those had proven infection (Table III). ^{111}In-granulocytes localized at infected sites in both patients. One patient had extensive oral ulcers and submandibular cellulitis and one had pneumonia demonstrable on chest X-ray. Four of 8 patients with both GC and LC antibodies had proven infections (Table III). Two patients had acute myelogeneous leukemia; one with extensive cellulitis of the thigh and one with

Table 3. Relationship of the results of indium body scans to granulocyte incompatibility determined by granulocyte agglutination (GA), granulocytotoxicity (GC) and lymphocytotoxicity (LC)*

Cross-match result[1] GA	GC	LC	Total studies	True-negative	True-positive	False-negative	False-positive
+	-	-	4	4	-	-	-
-	+	-	10	5	5	-	-
-	-	+	6	4	2	-	-
-	+	+	8	4	4	-	-
+	+	+	2	2	-	-	-
+[2]	+	-	1	-	-	1	-
+	-	+	1	-	-	1	-
-	-	-	26	11	12	-	3
Total			58	30	23	2	3

1) A minus indicates no reaction between recipient's serum and donor cells, and thus, indicates a compatible transfusion, while a plus indicates incompatibility.
2) The GA antibody in this patient was anti-NA1.

* From (20) with permission.

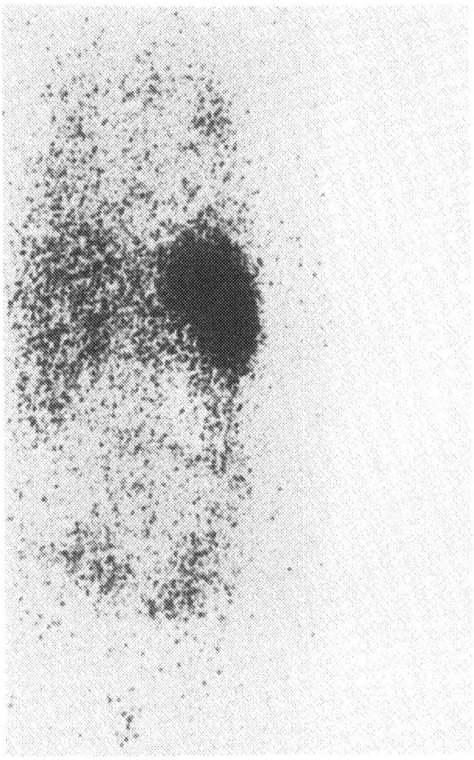

Figure 3. Indium-111 scan of 45-year-old female with acute myclogenous leukemia, pseudomembranous colitis, oral and anal ulcers. Despite the presence of a granulocytotoxic antibody that reacted with the donor's cells, there is accumulation of radioactivity in the mouth, lungs, right and left pelvis, and anal areas. (From (20) with permission).

pneumonia. The other 2 patients had pneumonia and rejection of a transplanted kidney. ^{111}In-granulocytes localized at all of these sites of infection (thighs, lungs, and kidney). Thus, 11 different patients with proven infection had localization of ^{111}In-granulocytes at the infected site (true-positive scan) in the presence of either GC or LC antibodies alone or in combination. Two other patients with proven infection did not show localization of ^{111}In-granulocytes at infected sites (false-negative scan), and both of these patients had GA antibodies (one combined with GC and one with LC).

Storage of granulocytes

Intravascular recovery and survival (22): Granulocytes from portions of five concentrates collected by leukaphersis were studied immediately after collection (Table IV). The average intravascular recovery was 30 ± 9% which is similar to our previous reported value of 31 ± 8% obselocytes studies of autologous granulocytes collected by phlebotomy (19). The half-life in the ciruclation of 2.5 ± 0.6 hours for unstored cells collected by leukapheresis is significantly less ($p < 0.01$) than the 5.0 ± 1.5 hours previously reported by us for granulocytes collected by phlebotomy.

Table 4. Effect of storage time and temperature on the intravascular kinetics and migration into skin windows of autologous ^{111}In-granulocytes in normal human subjects*

	Time (hours)	Temp.	N	Recovery %	Half-life (hours)	# Indium-111 cell/chamber	Migration ($x10^{-3}$)	Percent migration index
Phlebotomy	0		13	31 ± 8	5.0 ± 1.5	13500 ± 9500	25.0	
Leukapheresis	0		5	30 ± 0	2.5 ± 0.6	17500 ± 16800	19.0	3.09
	8	20-24°	4	28 ± 10	1.7 ± 0.6	8200 ± 6200	8.4	3.26
	8	1- 6°	4	10 ± 2[1,2]	1.8 ± 0.2	1250 ± 700	3.2[3,4]	0.38
	24	20-24°	5	15 ± 5[1]	3.0 ± 1.1	1500 ± 900[3]	2.5[3]	2.04[3]
	24	1- 6°	5	9 ± 2[1,2]	1.4 ± 0.4[1,2]	2000 ± 1400[3]	2.0[3]	1.48[3]

1) Values significantly less ($p < 0.03$) than comparable granulocytes not stored.
2) Value significantly less ($p < 0.05$) than granulocytes stored the same period of time at 20-24°C.
3) Values statistically significantly different ($p < 0.05$) from unstored granulocytes collected by leukapheresis.
4) Significantly different ($p < 0.05$) from cells stored 8 hours at 20–24°C.

* Adapted from (22) with permission.

When granulocytes were collected by leukapheresis and stored for 24 hours, the average intravascular recovery was significantly less ($p < 0.03$) than the percent recovery of unstored granulocytes regardless of the storage temperature (Table IV). In addition, the percent recovery of granulocytes stored at 20-24°C was significantly higher ($p < 0.05$) than for granulocytes stored at 1-6°C. The half-life of cells which circulated after storage for 24 hours (3.0 ± 1.1) was not different from unstored granulocytes collected by leukapheresis, and was significantly higher than for cells stored at 24 hours at 1-6°C (1.4 ± 0.4).

In 8 separate studies, granulocytes were stored for only 8 hours. The average intravascular recovery of granulocytes stored at 20-24°C (28 ± 10%) was not significantly different from unstored granulocytes collected by leukapheresis or phlebotomy and was significantly higher than granulocytes stored for 24 hours at 20-24°C (28 versus 15%; $p < 0.05$). Thus, the shorter storage period allowed maintenance of normal intravascular recovery. The half-life of granulocytes stored 8 hours at 20-24°C (1.7 ± 0.6 hours) was not different from fresh granulocytes collected by leukapheresis, but significantly lower than fresh cells collected by phlebotomy. After 8 hours storage at 1-6°C, the average recovery 11 ± 2%) was significantly less ($p < 0.05$) than unstored granulocytes. The half-life (1.9 ± 0.1 hours) was not different from fresh granulocytes or those stored 8 hours at 20-24°C.

Migration into skin windows (22): More important than the ability of stored granulocytes to circulate is their ability to migrate to sites of infection. Initially 13 subjects were studied to establish normal values for the skin window technique.

The skin window method used here is quite reproducible (mean of $52x10^6$ cells/chamber; range $37.3-80.7x10^6$), is not uncomfortable for the subject, gives a consistent area of exposed dermis and does not cause bleeding. The lesions are hyperpigmented for several weeks but none of the 34 subjects we have studied thus far has experienced scarring.

The inflammatory response of the subject is represented by the total number of leukocytes (indium-labeled and non-labeled) which migrate into the chambers during the 24 hours they are in place. This averaged 52 ± $13x10^6$ leukocytes per chamber. When granulocytes were collected by phlebotomy, labeled with indium-111 and injected immediately, there was an average of 13,500 ± 9,500 labeled cells recovered in the chambers. This represented $25x10^{-3}$% of the injected ^{111}In-granulocytes. When granulocytes were collected by leukapheresis and injected without storage, a similar number and percent of indium-111-labeled cells migrated into the chambers (Table IV). After storage for 24 hours at either 1-6°C or 20-24°C, there was significant reduction in the percent migration ($p < 0.005$) and the MI ($p < 0.025$). Granulocytes stored for 8 hours at 1-6°C also had significant reductions ($p < 0.05$) in the number and percent of cells migrating into the chambers and the MI. Despite the shorter storage time, these cells did not migrate better than cells stored 24 hours. However, shortening the storage time to 8 hours at 20-24°C resulted in improvement in the number and percent of ^{111}In-granulocytes which migrated into the chambers and the MI. None of these values were significantly different from unstored granulocytes. The difference in migration index between cells stored for 8 hours at 1-6°C and 20-24°C was statistically significant ($p < 0.05$).

DISCUSSION

The establishment of successful transfusion parameters is still one of the more difficult aspects concerning granulocyte transfusion. Methods of transfusion, dosage and frequency of administration appear to play some role in success (25). It is important to identify techniques that will help determine the effectiveness of such infusions. Studies of the kinetics of radio-labeled granulocytes have provided valuable information about their normal life span, mechanism of clearance from the circulation, and their extravascular location. The commercial unavailability of ^{32}DFP led to our investigations and subsequent use of inidum-111 as a useful substitute.

Indium-111-oxine labels granulocytes with high efficiency and appears to be firmly bound to the cell, since no elution or reutilization of the label has been demonstrated by the <u>in vitro</u> studies (19, 26). When an essentially pure granulocyte suspension is used, the injected radioactivity is either associated with the granulocytes or free in the supernatant solution. Consequently, manipulation of posttransfusion blood samples to determine granulocyte recovery and survival minimized, required only the substraction of plasma radioactivity from whole blood radioactivity. Previous <u>in vitro</u> studies of ^{111}In-granulocytes have shown normal viability, chemotaxis, bactericidal capacity, random migration, and oxygen consumption (19,27,28).

Our studies of granulocyte kinetics performed in ten normal volunteers showed a maximum intravascular recovery of 20 ± 5.9% of the ^{111}In-granulocytes injected. This level of recovery is somewhat lower than the normal recoveries reported using ^{32}DFP-labeled cells (40-50%) (2,29). The procedure used here for labeling granulocytes with ^{111}In requires more manipulations of the blood than does the DFP-labeling procedure. Thus, it is conceivable that the lower recovery observed in our study is a result of damage to the cells during the preparation, and this causes their immediate removal from the circulation following injection.

A valuable feature of ^{111}In is that it allows the use of scintigraphic techniques to study the fate of injected radio-labeled cells. The early distribution of radioactivity in the lungs, which we observed, has also been reported by Thakur et al. (30). In the absence of inflammation, this lung activity is rapidly cleared, and, subsequently, radioactivity appears predominantly in the liver and the spleen. Because normal uptake of radioactivity occurred mainly in these two areas, the presence of radioactivity in sites of inflammation or abscess was readily apparent.

^{111}In-granulocytes can also be used to study the effect of different variables, such as histocompatibility, in vivo chemotaxis, collection procedures, and storage conditions which may be important in the success of granulocyte transfusions.

Immunization of dogs by bloodtransfusion or skin grafting causes a reduced posttransfusion increment in granulocyte count (31,32). However, the serologic technique that most accurately reflects this immunization is not known (33). Usually a leukocyte rather than granulocyte suspension is used in the agglutination test, and the success of a granulocyte transfusion evaluated by the increase in count. These increases often average approximately $200/10^{10}$ granulocytes transfused/sq m body surface area (33), which in an infected neutropenic patient may not be a suitable endpoint because of patient variables and the error of the granulocyte count in that range. Despite the variables introduced by the patients in our study, the ^{111}In technique showed that GA antibodies altered the fate of granulocytes in vivo. Such alterations did not occur in the presence of GC or LC antibodies.

The use of the skin chamber provided a means of studying the in vivo chemotaxis in the absence of localized infection. The number of labeled granulocytes present in the chambers was a small percentage of the total leukocytes accumulated. However, the values seem reasonable when the number of labeled granulocytes injected is compared with the total granulocyte turnover in the subject over the 24-hour period. In addition to providing in vivo evidence of normal chemotaxis of ^{111}In-granulocytes, these results indicated that the labeled granulocytes, rather than secondarily labeled serum proteins, are responsible for most of the radioactivity at sites of inflammation or abscess.

Several reports have indicated that chemotactic response is reduced after storage of granulocytes but is better maintained by storage at 20-24°C than 1-6°C (17,34,36). Our studies indicate that the in vivo effectiveness of granulocytes stored for 24 hours is also decreased. The intravascular recovery was significantly reduced after 24 hours of storage at either temperature and after 8 hours of storage at 1-6°C. However, the percent migration and the MI were not significantly different from fresh granulocytes when granulocytes were stored at 20-24°C for 8 hours. The percent migration takes into consideration all cells including those not circulating after injection while the MI is based only on circulating cells. The percent migration is reduced by the influence of non-circulating cells although those that do circulate may migrate normally. The MI is reduced when there is impaired migration by the circulating cells. The data reported here suggest that storage reduces both the ability of cells to circulate and the ability of circulating cells to migrate to sites of inflammation. Although, shortening the storage interval to 8 hours and maintaining the granulocytes at 20-24°C produces cells that should be clinically effective.

Determining the efficacy of granulocyte transfusions depends not only on the condition and storage of the product from the donor, but also on variables inherent in the recipient. Criteria used to evaluate the clinical significance of these factors has varied from one institution to another and has been difficult to establish. Our experience has shown indium-labeled granulocytes are one tool which can be used to determine the in vivo effectiveness of granulocyte transfusions.

REFERENCES

1. Alexanian, R., Donahue, R.M. Neutrophilic granulocyte kinetics in normal man. J. App. Physiol. 1964;20:803–8.
2. Deinard, A.S., Page, A.R. An improved method for performing neutrophil survival studies. Blood 1970;36:98–100.
3. Mauer, A.M., Athens, J.W., Ashenbrucker, H., Cartwright, G.E., Wintrobe, M.M. Leukokinetic studies. II. A method for labeling granulocytes in vitro with radioactive diisopropylfluorophosphate (DFP-32). J. Clin. Invest. 1960;29:1481–6.
4. Dresch, C., Najean, Y., Bauchet, J. Kinetic studies of Cr-51 and DFP-32 labeled granulocytes. Br. J. Haematol. 1975;29: 67–80.
5. McMillan, R., Scott, J.L. Leukocyte labeling with chromium-51. I. Technique and results in normal subjects. Blood 1968;32: 738–54.
6. Thakur, M.L. Indium-111: A new radioactive tracer for leukocytes. Exp. Heamtol. 1977;5:145 (suppl.).
7. Thakur, M.L., Coleman, R.E., Welch, M.J. Indium-111-labeled leukocytes for the localization of abscesses: Preparation, analysis, tissue distribution, and comparison with gallium-67 citrate in dogs. J. Lab. Clin. Med. 1977;89:217–28.
8. McCullough, J., Clay, M.E., Priest, J.R. et al. A comparison of methods for detecting leukocyte antibodies in autoimmune neutropenia. Transfusion 1981;21:483–92.
9. Graw, R.G. Jr, Eyre, H.J., Goldstein, I.M., Terasaki, P.I. Histocompatibility testing for leukocyte transfusion. Lancet 1970;2:77–9.
10. Goldstein, I.M., Eyre, H.J., Terasaki, P.I., Henderson, E.S., Graw R.G. Jr. Leukocyte transfusions: Role of leukocyte alloantibodies in determining transfusion response. Transfusion 1971;11:19–24.
11. Eyre, H.J., Goldstein, I.M., Perry, S., Graw R.G. Jr. Leukocyte transfusion: Function of transfused granulocytes from donors with chronic myelocytic leukemia. Blood 1970;36:432–42.
12. McCredie, K.B., Hester, J.P., Freireich, E.J., Brittin, G.M., Vallejos, C. Platelet and leukocyte transfusions in acute leukemia. Human Pathol. 1974;5:699–708.
13. Schiffer, C.A., Buchholz, D.H., Aisner, J., Betts, S.W., Wiernik, P.H. Clinical experience with transfusions of granulocytes obtained by continuous flow filtration leukapheresis. Am. J. Med. 1975;58:373–81.

14. McCullough, J., Wood, N., Weiblen, B.J., Fortuny, I.E., Yunis, E.J. The role of histocompatibility testing in granulocyte transfusion. In: Greenwalt, T.J., Jamieson, G.A. (eds.) The Granulocyte: Function and clinical utilization. New York: Alan R. Liss, 1977, pp. 321–7.
15. McCullough, J. Liquid preservation of granulocytes. Transfusion 1980;20:129–37.
16. Price, R.H., Dale, D.C. Blood kinetics and in vivo chemotaxis of transfused neutrophils: Effect of collection method, donor corticosteroid treatment and short-term storage. Blood 1979;54:977–86.
17. McCullough, J., Weiblen, G.J., Peterson, P.K., Deinard, A.S., Quie, P.G. Effects of temperature on granulocyte preservation. Blood 1978;52:301–10.
18. Palm, S.L., Furcht, L.T., McCullough, J. Effects of temperature and duration of storage on granulocyte adhesion, spreading, and ultrastructure. Lab. Invest. 1981;45:82–8.
19. Weiblen, B.J., Forstrom, K., McCullough, J. Studies of the kinetics of indium-111-labeled granulocytes. J. Lab. Clin. Med. 1979;94:246–55.
20. McCoullough, J., Weiblen, B.J., Clay, M.E., Forstrom, L. Effect of leukocyte antibodies on the fate in vivo of indium-111-granulocytes. Blood 1981;58:164–70.
21. Terasaki, P.I, Park, M.S. Microdroplet lymphocyte cytotoxicity test. Bethesda, MD: NIAID Manual of Tissue Typing Techniques, 1976. (DHEW publication No. (NIH) 77545), pp. 69–85.
22. McCoullough, J., Weiblen, B.J., Fine, D. Effects of storage of granulocytes on their fate in vivo. Transfusion (in press).
23. Weiblen, B.J., McCoullough, J., Forstrom, K., Loken, M.K. Kinetics of Indium-111-labeled granulocytes. In: Thakur, M.L., Gottschalk, A. (eds.) Indium-111-labeled neutrophils, platelets and lymphocytes. Proceedings of the Yale symposium on radio-labeled cellular elements. New York, Trivirum, 1980, pp. 23–32.
24. Loken, M.K., Forstrom, L.A., Cook, A., McCoullough, J. 111-Indium-labeled leukocytes for diagnosing inflammatory diseases of the abdomen and neutrophil space. In: Wahner, H.W., Goodwin, D.A. (eds.) Cell labeling and imaging procedures with indium-111. Proceedings of the second annual workshop on platelet and lekuocyte labeling, Mayo Clinic, Rochester, Minnesota, 1981. Crystal Lake, Illinois: Central Chapter Society of Nuclear Medicin (in press).
25. Higby, D., Burnett, D. Granulocyte transfusions: Current status. Blood 1980;55:2–8.
26. Thakur, M.L., Segal, A.W., Louis, L., Welch, M.J., Hopkins, J., Peters, T.J. Indium-111-labeled cellular blood components: Mechanism of labeling and intracellular location in human neutrophils. J. Nucl. Med. 1977;18:1022–6.
27. Segal, A.W., Deteix, P, Garcia, R., Tooth, P., Zanelli, G.D., Allison, A.C. Indium-111-labeling of leukocytes: A detrimental effect on neutrophil and lymphocyte function and an improved method of cell labeling. J. Nucl. Med. 1978;19:1238–44.

28. Zakhireh, B., Thakur, M.L., Maleck, H.L., Cohen, M.S., Gottschalk, A., Root, R.K. Indium-111-labeled human polymorphonuclear leukocytes: Viability, random migration, chemotaxis, bactericidal capacity, and ultrastructure. J. Nucl. Med. 1979;20:741–7.
29. Price, T.H., Dale, D.C. Neutrophil transfusion: Effect of storage and collection method on neutrophil kinetics. Blood 1978;51:789–98.
30. Thakur, M.L., Lavender, J.P., Arnot, R.M., Silvester, D.J., Segal, A.W. Indium-111-labeled autologous leukocytes in man. J. Nucl. Med. 1977;18:1014–21.
31. Westrick, M.A., Debelak-Fehir, K.M., Epstein, R.B. The effect of prior whole blood transfusion on subsequent granulocyte support in leukopenic dogs. Transfusion 1977;17:611–207.
32. Appelbaum, F.R., Trapani, R.J., Graw, R.G. Jr. Consequences of prior alloimmunization during granulocyte transfusion. Transfusion 1977;17:460–4.
33. Ungerleider, R.S., Appelbaum, F.R., Trapani, R.J., Deisseroth, A.B. Lack of predictive value of antileukocyte antibody screening in granulocyte transfusion therapy. Transfusion 1979;19:90–4.
34. Glasser, L. The effect of storage on normal neutrophils collected by discontinuous-flow centrifugation leukapheresis. Blood 1977;50:1145–50.
35. Steigbiegl, R.T., Baum, J., MacPherson, J.L., Nusbacher, J. Granulocyte, bactericidal capacity, and chemotaxis as affected by continuous-flow centrifugation and filtration leukapheresis, steroid administration and storage. Blood 1978;52: 197–109.

DISCUSSION

Moderators: M.R. Halie, Ch.A. Schiffer

J.A. van der Does, 's Gravenhage, The Netherlands:

I would like to make a comment on the presentation of Dr. Sintnicolaas about the prevention of urticarial reactions in patients. He proposes to wash the cells for these patients. I think that a lot of patients do not always get those reactions on subsequent transfusions. As washing is a tedious procedure, I do not think that washing for that indication is to be recommended.

K. Sintnicolaas, Rotterdam, The Netherlands:

When patients have repeated reactions, there are two ways to prevent them. The first one is to give antihistamines before transfusion. Secondly, when they still have reactions, then one should use washed cells.

J.A. van der Does:

May I ask a question to Dr. de Beus on the disconnection-proof transfusion system? I agree upon a patient with chronic anaemia, who comes in for his weekly or bi-weekly transfusion. But, the acutely ill patient in the hospital, who needs a lot of blood, requires much changing of infusion solutions. The nurse changes the infusion quite a number of times. To devote so much attention to the disconnection-proof of the whole system is not warranted in those situations. The intravenous catheter for giving infusions which can last for days, weeks or even months with the jugular or sub-clavian catheters is, I think a good practice for critically ill patients. I agree with you that this is a minor surgical operation to insert them, but these catheters will save the patient a lot of pain from repeated veini-punctures.

H. de Beus, Assen, The Netherlands:

There may be some misunderstanding. When I am speaking of a disconnection-proof system, I am referring to a mechanical point of view. In the olden days when we were using glass bottles, the needle from an administration set had to be pierced through the rubber. Most of us have seen patients, especially in the surgical department or in operating theaters, with a disconnected system. A bag and spike system provides a stable and safe connection. Thus, we are talking about different questions. We have touched on the possibility of extrinsic contamination by invasion of the transfusion system. One has to reflect on how many invasions can be made into the infusion channel! I have tried to describe this in the mechanical way. Considering the microbiological way, figures from the literature are very significant. One of the reasons that thrombophlebitis incidence is high, especially in those departments of the hospital like coronary care and intensive care units, but also in the ward, is that there are many invasions via injections into the intravenous chain. This should be prevented as much as possible.

Ch.A. Schiffer:

I would support that. My interest is in the management of severely myelo-suppressed patients. In our unit, the rule is if the patient has a scalp-vein needle, it is reinserted every 24 hours. We see virtually no local cellulitis or thrombophlebitis. This is in contast to practice at many other hospitals. Of course, it is an inconvenience to be "stuck" frequently, but what we attempt to do is to combine that with the time that the patient would have blood drawn. To some extend this has been replaced by indwelling Hickman-type catheters, but nonetheless when you are using standard catheters, it is important to replace them frequently.

W.L. Marsh, New York, USA:

I would like to comment on Dr. Reesink's excellent presentation. My comment refers to the need that has been stressed so repeatedly in this meeting: We must continuously revise and re-evaluate the procedures and the thinking that we follow.

Among the list of parasitic diseases that you gave us was babesiosis. Until a few years ago it was virtually unknown as a transmittable disease. At the moment in Northeast America, babesiosis is a problem of significant proportions. Until a few years ago, the disease was restricted to a few of the islands offshore. It has now reached such proportions that the local health authorities felt that they should warn all visitors to the islands that the disease existed. It is transmitted by thick bite, but has now spread, and is present in the islands at the end of Long Island, in Connecticut and Massachusetts. There are a number of deaths reported from babesiosis – all of these patients have been splenectomized. We no longer collect blood at the end of Long Island because of the risk of babesiosis. So, all of us have to continually re-evaluate how we approach diseases which we thought were rare and virtually non existent. Perhaps there are changing profils. Babesiosis concerns us.

Ch.A. Schiffer:

Since we are mentioning unusual things, it might be of interest to say that there have now been three cases of the acquired immune deficiency syndrome in patients with hemophilia in the United States. These are patients who are all using a great deal of AHF. The concern is that this is no longer found simply either in the gay population or the Haitian population. It tells us potentially something about the transmissibility of that disease. Do you have a comment?

W.L. Marsh:

Can I just add a rider to my comment? I meant to mention that one of the posttranfusion deaths in a splenectomized patient was caused by transmission of babesiosis, the unit of blood had been collected and been stored in glycerol, deep-frozen for some months before it was transfused, and yet it still transmitted babesiosis.

J. Leikola, Geneva, Switzerland:

I am a bit troubled by the question of non-A non-B hepatitis, especially the high figures that are generally given for the chronic form of the disease after transfusion. If we assume that there are about 11 million units of blood collected annually in the United States, it was said that about 3-4% of the units are infective for non-A non-B hepatitis. If we assume that there are something like 10-12 million transfusions in the United States, including platelet, fresh frozen plasma and so forth, then we would end up with a figure of over 400,000 transfusions of hepatitis non-A non-B per year. Of these 200,000 would be of a chronic nature, if it is assumed that about 40% of those cases lead to a chronic disease. Assuming that 10-20% of the acute cases are icteric, there should be around 40,000-80,000 icteric cases of non-A non-B posttransfusion hepatitis per year in the United States. Some statistics indicate that there are altogether 100,000 reported cases of infectious hepatitis per year in the United States and only a small minority are posttranfusion hepatitis. I would like to have some comments on this epidemiology from the American colleagues.

H.W. Reesink, Amsterdam, The Netherlands:

It is a major concern in the United States, so perhaps my collegues from the USA can comment on this later. The fact that the reported cases are always behind the actual cases found in prospective studies, is why the prospective studies are so important. Cases of sub-clinical hepatitis, especially of the non-A non-B type, are not mentioned in the reported cases. Most of these chronic hepatitis cases are asymptomatic. It is like the HBsAg carrier state. No one knows what is going on. In Europe far less non-A non-B hepatitis is found. In The Netherlands, a remarkable study was done by Katchaki*, describing thirteen patients with non-A non-B hepatitis, all had normal liver functions after six months. So, at least these thirteen cases did not develop into chronic disease.

H.F. Taswell, Rochester, USA:

I do not think we have enough information to make the calculation Dr. Leikola just went through. For example, there is one important piece of information missing. We do not know the prevalence of the antibody in the population. For example, for anti-hepatitis B, depending on the population and the age group, 30-50% of the people being transfused may have the antibody. We have no idea of what the prevalence of an antibody for the non-A non-B hepatitis is. So apparently a lot of those people transfused, primarily in the older age group, are protected. When we talk about chronic non-A non-B hepatitis, we are talking about a whole spectrum of disease from the asymptomatic carrier through benign persistent hepatitis all the way to severe chronic active liver disease. Another factor is that chronic means more than six months with elevated enzymes. You could have someone who had this for seven or eight months, then it disappears and they are well. So, all of those things would have to be factored into it before we could come to a real answer.

J.G. Eernisse, Leiden, The Netherlands:

I would like to comment on Dr. Beus' lecture. The laboratory which does the cross-matching and orders the blood from the blood bank was not included at all in the considerations regarding transfusions. As far as I am concerned, they are very important in all the decision making for transfusions in the patients. Usually the doctor is some kind of god, and he orders for delivery at inconvenient times of the day without concern about what the laboratory can do and has to do. In good hospital practice, anything these non-clinical workers have to add to the transfusion procedure must be taken into consideration. Another aspect is the transfusion history of the patients. The blood transfusion laboratory records all the transfusion requests and transfusion reactions are registered there as well. I think that a major part of the whole transfusion service in the hospital goes through this clinical laboratory. All the information stored there should not be ignored.

H. de Beus:

I fully agree with your comment. But my intention was to make a plea that good manufacturing practice outside the hospital should continue on the same level inside the hospital. The complexity of good hospital practice consists of two parts. Good laboratory

* Katchaki, J.N. et al. J. Vir. Meth. 1980;2:119–25.

practice is number one. It is certainly not the final step to the total transfusion procedure from vein to vein.

I have restricted myself to the second part of good hospital practice, the clinical part, which is the responsibility of the clinician. In our hospital the position of the laboratory was difficult in the days when – as it perhaps still is in your hospital – the request for blood by surgical team came too late in the day. It must be scheduled earlier.

W.L. Marsh:

Could I ask Dr. Reesink's views on the value of ALT screening in trying to detect the non-A non-B hepatitis carriers? In New York, in the last year, we have been screening on an automated procedure all donors for ALT. We lose approximately 2% of the donors. I understand the cost per test is about just a fraction over $1.

H.W. Reesink:

As you know, this is questioned everywhere. I think the policy of your country, following the advice of a special committee, is not to test for ALT at this moment. There are more arguments against it than in favour of it. The policy elsewhere in the world is roughly the same at this moment, although several countries, like the Federal Republic of Germany and Luxemburg, were screening for ALT for 25 years. The general opinion at the moment is to await the specific test for non-A non-B hepatitis, and not to test for ALT. This opinion may change when more data are available.

W.L. Marsh:

The real question, of course, is whether you can reduce the incidence of non-A non-B by doing a screening of this kind. Despite the discussion that goes on among many eminent authorities, the only way to find out is to do it. That is why we decided that we would do it. There have been screened about 400,000 people at the moment. We do not as yet have the data, but we hope that in the near future we will have data to show whether it has reduced the incidence at all.

Ch.A. Schiffer:

Is this a randomized study?

W.L. Marsh:

Every single donor coming through is tested.

Ch.A. Schiffer:

Is the blood rejected; or is it transfused?

W.L. Marsh:

It is rejected.

Ch.A. Schiffer:

I can anticipate the criticism of your results.

A.C.J.M. Holdrinet, Breda, The Netherlands:

I have a question for Dr. Reesink. There is a suggestion in the literature that hepatitis B virus and non-A non-B share the core system. Can you comment on that and on the testing for antibodies against hepatitis core antigen. That presumably reduces the incidence of posttransfusion hepatitis.

H.W. Reesink:

That is difficult to answer. Some studies in the United States on donors having this core antibody have shown an increased incidence of posttransfusion hepatitis B, as well as non-A non-B hepatitis. The purpose of Katchaki's study* in The Netherlands was to show the significance of the anti-core antibody in donors. In this study he compared the donations of about 180 donors with anti-HBc with a control group of donors without anti-HBc; the patients were prospectively followed-up. He found three hepatitis B cases in the anti-HBc positive group versus zero in the control group. Although, these data were not significant, there may be a trend towards the anti-HBc group, in respect to posttranfusion hepatitis B. On the other hand, he did not find an excess of non-A non-B hepatitis cases in the anti-HBc group compared to the control group. That does not fit with the American data. However, it is still an open question. Screening for anti-HBc is a very costly affair. The data available now are too scarce to make a recommendation to screen all donors for anti-HBc.

Ch.A. Schiffer:

I guess the association is that the same type of donor who might contract one disease might contract the other, rather than it being a specific marker.

We also did studies of histocompatibility, using indium labeled granulocytes. There is no tool worth a darn to help you understand what you were doing after a granulocyte transfusion. Because of this, people totally ingnored histocompatibility factors

* Katchaki, J.N. et al.: Brit. Med. J. 1981;282:107–8.

when selecting donors for granulocyte transfusions. We began our studies a little bit later than the group in Minnesota. They were done predominantly by Dr. Dutcher from our group.

As reported in this meeting, we did a similar thing, except we did not do granulocyte kinetics, and did not use as clean a product as the Minnesota group. We chose patients who had obviously infections at sites that were away from the liver and the spleen, because the liver and the spleen will have radioactivity normally.

We used 10^8 granulocytes, separated by gravity sedimentation. We did not do kinetics, so we had to do something different. A computer was used to analyse the events spread over a period of time. What the computer does is to grade the degree of intensity of radiation, with blue being the least intense, red and yellow being the most intense. Our experimental design was similar. The hypothesis is: If a cell got to a site of infection, it was more likely to be a successful transfusion. If there was no radioactivity at the site of infection, it is highly unlikely that transfusion, if it would have been administered, would have been effective.

We studied a group of twenty non-alloimmunized patients, all of whom had identifiable infections. What does that mean? These were patients who respond to random donor platelets, and had no HL-A antibody. In twenty out of twenty the scan was positive when it should have been, meaning that the technique we used was a reliable one. None of these patients had lymphocytotoxic antibody and all of the cross-matches that were done were negative. Three patients had a positive leuko-agglutinin cross-match. I am not certain what that means, but at any event the scans were positive despite that.

A second group were alloimmunized patients who in contrast had HL-A antibody and were clearly refractory to random-donor platelets. This very heavily alloimmunized group of patients was deliberately selected. This is somewhat different than the initial group studied in Minnesota. A total of fourteen patients were studied, eleven had negative scans in contrast to twenty out of twenty patients in the previous study. This is obviously statistically highly significant. Almost all of them had positive lymphocytotoxic cross-matches, and most had positive leuko-agglutin cross-matches as well. There were three exceptions to the rule, and it was interesting that in two out of three the scans were positive despite alloimmunization. Fortuitously all the donors, who were laboratory personnel, were HL-A compatible, if not identical with the recipient.

The conclusions of this study, in parallel with the other, are that alloimmunization adversely and severely affects the migration of granulocytes to sites of infections, and hence almost certainly affects the clinical results of such transfusions. How it translates into practice is: Usually we attempt to use compatible platelet donors for such patients, but if we do not have what we think might be a compatible donor, we will not give them granulocytes, simply because we think there is overwhelming evidence that those transfusions are likely to be ineffective. What we cannot say is which antibody is important. Alloimmunized leukemic patients tend to have multiple types of antibodies simultaneously. Our data, and perhaps the Minnesota data as well, do not precisely say which type of cross-match would be preferable. But it is also quite clear that alloimmunization is a very important factor in granulocyte transfusion. It is really one that clinicians and blood bankers can no longer ignore.

M.R. Halie:

May I call on Dr. Eernisse to give his comments on the alloimmunization in platelets and the harvesting of platelets without leukocytes form random non-matched donors?

J.G. Eernisse:

It is difficult to comment on Dr. Sintnicolaas' paper. If patients have been transfused with red cells containing leukocytes, and by platelets containing leukocytes, you may end up by having to do a platelet apheresis on a matched donor. Alternatively, you can start supporting the patient by selected apheresis, which we would not like. This is a costly program, because these donors have to be typed and stored in a computer. Some donors leave the Blood Transfusion Centre over the years requiring a constant recruiting. In 1976 we had 34 new patients who had to be transfused, with a matched donor, while we had started giving leukocyte free preparations in 1974. We expected the figures to keep rising with every leukemia patient needing matched donor platelets, but things changed. The number decreased. At the moment, we have not given any matched platelets during the first half of 1982, despite a potential of matched donors. Not having to do platelet apheresis is indeed a great saving. The cost-benefit is enormous. Over 1973-1974 we had about 2,000 random platelet transfusions. At the moment, it is well over 8,000.

P. Rebulla, Milan, Italy:

Dr. Schiffer's study was a very nice study. We are trying to repeat it in a slightly different way, technically. We developed in our blood bank a simple system to get rid of virtually all leukocytes in the platelet preparation. This consists of filtering them through the Terumo IG-500 filters. We expect that refractoriness to random platelet concentrates could be delayed if we adopt a policy of leukocyte-free blood components (red cells and platelet concentrates) for patients who are at risk of developing refractoriness. Leukocyte-poor blood components would be not enough poor.

K. Sintnicolaas:

I want to reply to Dr. Eernisse's comment: Why did we try single apheresis donors? We agree that it is valuable to test methods to decrease alloimmunization, and there were several options. You choose for the method using leukocyte depleted platelets. We have choosen to do it by single donor transfusion, because that is an other option. Although it has been suggested by others that this could work, no data are available. We therefore took that option to see whether indeed it would work. When both methods work, I think the cost-benefit ratio will determine which is to be used preferably. Perhaps your method is more convenient to use, but I think it is valuable to study whether single donor platelet concentrates really will decrease alloimmunization.

Ch.A. Schiffer:

I agree with Dr. Sintnicolaas. I think you are asking a very important biological question. It is one which will probably be very difficult to implement, should your study prove positive. It is an important question for a number of reasons, but it certainly is not one that should be done by anyone who is not studying it. I do not know why our observations seem to be different from yours, Dr. Eernisse. I doubt whether the major factor is the frozen red cells. I suspect it has something to do with the platelets. We were unable to get as profound a lymphocyte depletion as you, except that I believe the number of $1x10^8$ per unit of platelet concentrate is pretty low. It is about as low as we have been able to get without losing substantial numbers of platelets. We are not familiar with Japanese filters. I think for patients with leukemia, which is the largest group of patients whom I care for, the arithmetic that I went through at the end of my talk is still an important question, and it is one we are all going to have to address if we are successful in getting each other to believe that one method or another is pretty sure to prevent alloimmunization.

Dr. Halie asked a very important question as well: Do we all use the same definition of alloimmunization? It is very important that one utilizes a serologic definition as much as possible. One of the problems that Dr. Sintnicolaas showed in his clinical evaluation of alloimmunization was that you notice that at the first tranfusion of patients some of the single donor platelets did not work. But, with a second transfusion they did work. Hence it appeared that the results remained stable or actually improved from transfusion to transfusion. That probably has to do simply with the biological variability of these patients. It occurs in these patients all the time, from transfusion to transfusion. The best end point of that study, and of any study, is serology. Serology should not just be done once, it should be done repeatedly towards the end of induction therapy, a four to eight week periods in patients with acute leukemia.

What serology? We think that the simplest and most reproducible serology is lymphocytotoxicity. Because we have been able to demonstrate a very good correlation between lymphocytotoxicity and refractoriness to platelets, not against a donor, but just against a panel of donors. That is, about 90% of people who have reasonable levels of lymphocytotoxic antibody are refractory, i.e. have poor count increments. And the converse is true: about 90% who do not have antibody are not refractory. This will be published shortly.

J.A. Loos, Amsterdam, The Netherlands:

The number of leukocytes in platelet preparations can be made very low, if you use the method which is routinely used in Amsterdam. This is to prepare them from the buffy coat. We end up in the blood bank with numbers of 0.05×10^8 to 0.2×10^8. This is the average of about a thousand of units, I think.

Ch.A. Schiffer:

We had 0.1×10^8, obviously lower than your upper figure of 0.2×10^8. Our leukocyte-poor platelets, as I showed the data, were in the range you are talking about.

J.A. Loos:

The other thing is that all your data about platelets are based on platelets which have been stored in plasma. The method which is used in America is based on the fact that you first make platelet rich plasma and then concentrate the platelets by a second spin. The method developed by Prins* in 1976 is based on first making a buffy coat, spinning the platelets on top of the red cells, and during a second spin preparing platelet rich plasma from that buffy coat. In this way, you have concentrated the platelets but you have never aggregated them during production. If you store buffy coats with the platelets at 4°C, you will find after three days that platelets still can be aggregated with 1.6 micrograms of ADP per milliliter.

Another thing I want to comment on is the fact that you used the term osmotic shock response. Osmotic shock response can be calculated in very different ways. One of the most common methods is looking for osmotic shock response after 15 minutes. But you have to look at it kinetically, as was described by Odink**. Would you comment on that?

Ch.A. Schiffer:

I am rather more interested in the first comment. This is the first time it was explained to me how in Amsterdam platelets are

* Prins, H.K. et al. Med. et Hyg. 1980;38:1902–3.
** Odink, J. Thromb. and Haemost. 1976;36:182–91.

produced from buffy coat. To me it appears to be terribly cumbersome. What distrubs me most about it, is the necessity for storage at 4°C. I think that the data are overwhelming that 4°C storage severely compromises platelet survival. That is something that has been found in every study that has been published so far.

The comment about whether or not platelets aggregate to ADP is entirely accurate. Except, I am not sure it has any relevance to what happens in clinical practice. However, you are absolutely right, platelets stored at room temperature do not aggregate even with high concentrations of ADP. Nonetheless, they have normal survival, recovery and hemostatic functions. There is something that occurs posttransfusion which rectifies that defect. They do aggregate if you use a couple of aggregating agents simultaneously. What disturbs me potentially about that method of preparation is the necessity for storage at 4°C. I would like to see the data published.

H.F. Taswell:

As Chairman, I would like to interrupt. The papers that were presented are excellent, fascinating papers, and so is the discussion. But it is centering primarily on production of an ideal platelet preparation, or granulocyte preparation. This is, of course, very important. However, the symposium is a symposium on quality control. The technique such as indium labeling is a means that we hope will provide eventually a way of in vivo evaluation. There are other techniques for in vitro evaluation which apply to platelets, or granulocytes, or Factor VIII. Perhaps we could shift the discussion to these techniques or others and their application to in vitro and in vivo evaluations as quality control tool. Are they efficient? Are they usable now? Are they cost effective? How would one go about using these quality control tools?

C.F. Högman, Uppsala, Sweden:

I have a question and a comment to Dr. Schiffer, which relates to at least quality. It concerns the way of preparing platelets by centrifugation. People quite often do not define their manner of centrifugation well enough. This is particularly true if you have very brief centrifugation times, because then sufficient notice of the acceleration phase and the retardation phase is not taken. There recently was published a short paper in Vox Sanguinis* on this subject.

I have one more remark. This is about transfusing platelets. You did not mention anything about the transfusion set, when you give platelets to the patient. This is the very last part of the chain. Have you any comments on how to obtain a maximum yield in the patient?

* Högman, C.F. et al. Vox Sang. 1982;43:266–69.

Ch.A. Schiffer:

We just use a standard blood filter. I believe that is what most people use, but it should be a clean and saline primed filter.

R.E. de Vries, Enschede, The Netherlands:

It is not often that I apply indium labeled granulocytes in patients, but I transfuse platelets daily stored at 4°C, which now worries me!

J.A. Loos:

First of all, our method is not cumbersome, because routine production of buffy coats is much easier than routine production of platelet rich plasma. With respect to the storage conditions, you should bear in mind some data in the recent literature about the effect of oxygen on platelet survival (Murphy*), so one of the worst things you can do to platelets is to deprive them during storage from the red cells which are the source of oxygen in blood. Not only the oxygen transport capacity of red cells but also their ability to reduce oxidants and bind carbon monoxyde can help to protect the platelets against oxidative damage and acidification. As soon as you store platelets with red cells present, you have an enormous buffer of oxygen present. As soon as you start storing platelets in plasma alone and measure the oxygen tension, a very rapid fall of the oxygen tension is found in that plasma, because there is no buffer capacity left. I think this is the main difference. If you are talking about storage at 4°C, you mean storage in plasma. And this is not the same as storage in the presence of red cells. So, the ultimate thing that you should compare is the storage of platelets in whole blood in comparison to that in plasma.

Ch.A. Schiffer:

I do not think we are going to settle all the questions that we have addressed. However, I think the five-day bags are going to increase the quality of platelets considerably, because of their gas-exchange capacity and effect on oxygen tension. Of course, the issue of leukocytes will still remain. We are talking about the most important aspects of quality control. That is, what happens in the patient? We have all addressed things which may or may not be measurable in vitro. We have a very fundamental difference here about what is the best for patients. We happen to disagree, but I think that represents the ultimate issue in quality control and that is something that ought not to be ignored.

* Murphy, S., Holme, S. Transfusion 1981;21:637–38 (abstract).

V. Error analysis

ERROR ANALYSIS: TYPES OF ERRORS IN THE BLOOD BANK

H.F. Taswell, C.L. Sonnenberg

INTRODUCTION

As early as 1963, the importance of errors in blood banking was recognized by Schmidt (1). In a study of 5806 units of blood transfused at his hospital, he noted an error rate of 1 in 100 transfusions. Subsequently, a remarkably varying range of errors has been reported. In 1966, Kwa (2) reported only 1 error in 2000 transfusions. In contrast, Lacerte (3) reported an error rate of 1 in 3. In 1973, in our earliest study (4) of over 62,000 units transfused at the Mayo Clinic, we found an error rate of 1 in 500 units. Because these reports of widely varying error rates were all retrospective studies of errors which happened to have come to the attention of the management of the blood bank, it is difficult to evaluate their accuracy.

A more recent study by Schmidt (5,6) has emphasized the relationship between blood bank errors and transfusion mortality. Under the Freedom of Information Act in the United States, blood banking errors associated with transfusion mortality (which must be reported to the U.S. Government's Food and Drug Administration) are available to the public for study. In his review of 69 of these reports, Schmidt found that approximately one third of transfusion deaths reported to the Food and Drug Administration in 1976 to 1978 were associated with clerical error, the single most important cause of death in modern transfusion medicine. In a similar study of a larger number of these reports, Bove (7) found that 44% of these deaths were associated with hemolysis, usually due to an ABO incompatibility resulting from an error. Of these errors, 7 were related to collection and ordering of the blood sample, 13 occurred within the blood bank laboratory and 17 were due to improper administration of blood. In a third study of these reports over a longer period of time (1976-1979) Myhre (8) found that over 60% of the reported transfusion deaths were due to some type of clerical error. It is apparent from these studies, that currently the most significant cause of transfusion morbidity and mortality is human error. It is not due to our failure to recognize an anty-Fy^a or an anti-Kell, but, to our failure to do something as simple and unscientific as giving a

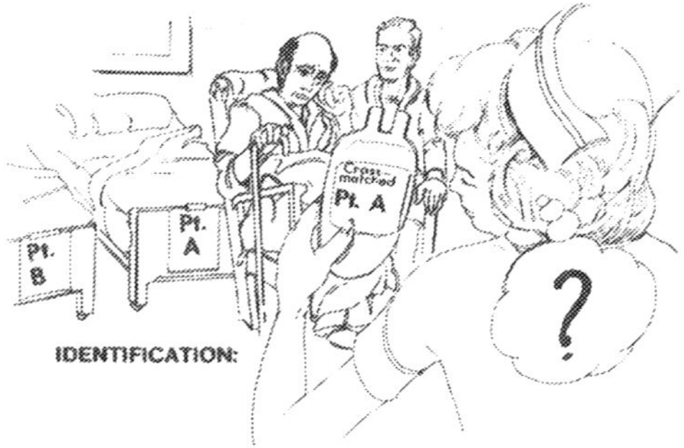

Figure 1.

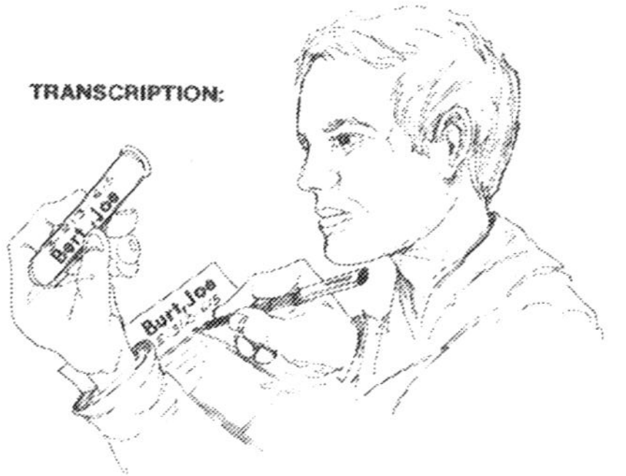

Figure 2.

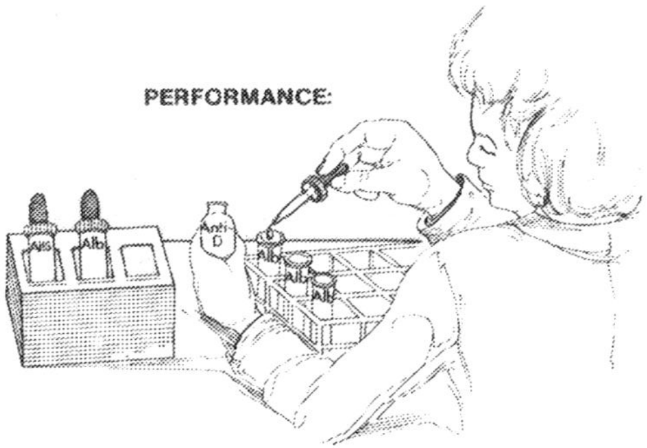

Figure 3.

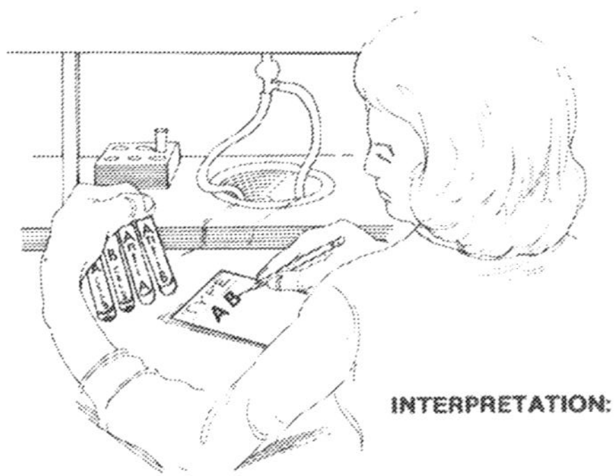

Figure 4.

blood transfusion to the correct patient or crossmatching the corrent sample of blood. Human error has now been clearly recognized as a significant cause of transfusion morbidity and mortality. A reduction in error rates will be achieved only after we acquire knowledge of the type and frequency of errors and respond with appropriate action.

FUNCTIONAL CLASSIFICATION

In a new and more studied approach to this problem (9), our initial objective was to classify all blood bank errors by function rather than by the traditional classification of errors as 'technical' or 'clerical'. We found these terms not to be useful since they do not define the problem adequately. Our specific objectives were to 1) develop a functional classification of all blood bank errors, 2) determine the frequency of blood bank errors, and 3) to evaluate the usefulness of this method of error analysis. To achieve these objectives, it was necessary that all errors occurring in the blood bank be identified, reported and recorded. These errors could then be analyzed and their frequency calculated in terms of both procedure and function. In addition, the reliability of error identification and reporting was monitored by the use of intentional errors that were sprinkled throughout the blood bank. When several thousand errors had been identified and analyzed, they were classified into one of five types of function carried out in the blood bank. These five types of blood bank functions which are prone to error include: 1) Identification (Fig. 1) of a patient, unit of blood or blood sample. 2) Performance (Fig. 2) of a myriad of different types of physical activity such as taking serum out of an anti-D reagent bottle and putting the proper number of drops into the proper tube. 3) Transcription (Fig. 3) of literally thousands of items of information which must be transferred from one piece of paper or object to another. 4) Interpretation (Fig. 4) of a pattern of test results, which must first be observed and then, a correct conclusion recorded. Another

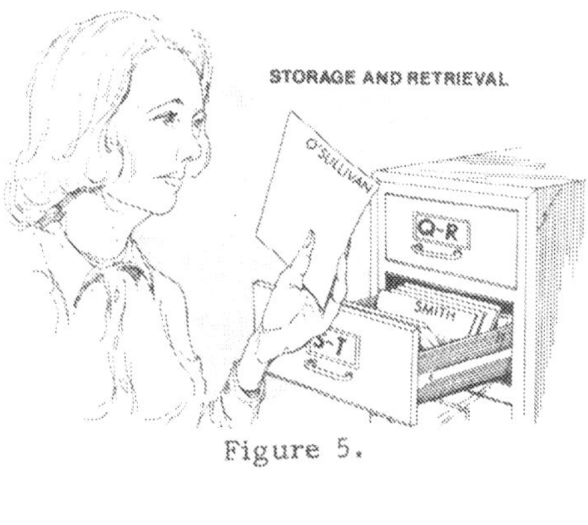

Figure 5.

function was recognized which we originally called Filing but soon realized should more appropriately be referred to as 5) Storage and Retrieval (Fig. 5) since it requires both the initial storage of clinically vital information, as well as its later rapid retrieval.

ERROR FREQUENCY: BY FUNCTION AND PROCEDURE

To determine error frequency by these newly defined functions, or by procedure, it is necessary to analyze the various services and procedures carried out within the blood bank which are critical to the safety of the patient. Such an analysis leads to the functional classification of each step in the procedure and therefore the frequency of each function within each procedure. The standard procedure for ABO/Rh typing (see Fig. 3 in the next Chapter) can be analyzed step by step. In our blood bank, we found that this procedure included 6 steps of identification, 11 steps of performance, 4 of interpretation, etc. Each procedure or service of critical importance to the patient's safety was analyzed similarly. In a period of 18 months, over 100,000 ABO/Rh typings were performed in our blood bank. In that time period, therefore, our laboratory technicians performed 743,000 identifications, 500,000 interpretations, etc. (Table I). When this approach was applied to all critical procedures in the blood bank, it became apparent that, between all blood bank personnel, 7.5 million identifications took place in those 18 months, as well as 12 million steps of performance, 7 million transcriptions, etc. (Table I). For the determination of the frequency of errors by function, these numbers serve as denominators since they are a measure of the frequency with which a particular function was performed. The number of times a functional error occurred (Table II) serves as the numer-

Tabel I. Blood bank procedures and frequency of function.

Function	Frequency of Function			
	ABO/Rh Type		All Procedures	
	By Test	In 18 months	By Test	In 18 months
Identification	6	743,703	265	7,522,334
Performance	11	1,302,021	417	11,911,116
Transcription	7	884,653	287	6,845,488
Interpretation	4	501,440	4	501,440
Storage & retrieval	2	522,534	2	522,534
Total	30	3,954,351	975	27,302,912

Table II. Blood bank errors: Identified by function (in 18 months).

Function	ABO/Rh Type	All Procedures
Identification	1	195
Performance	14	585
Transcription	11	842
Interpretation	3	3
Storage & retrieval	873	873
Total	902	2498

Table III. Blood bank errors: Frequency by function (in 18 months).

	%
Identification	$0.003 = \frac{195}{7,522,334}$
Performance	$0.005 = \frac{585}{11,911,116}$
Transcription	$0.012 = \frac{842}{6,845,448}$
Interpretation	$0.0006 = \frac{3}{501,440}$
Storage & retrieval	$0.17 = \frac{873}{522,634}$

Numerator: Sum of all errors within function.
Denominator: Sum of frequency of all functions in all procedures.

ator and provides, for the first time, a meaningful measure of error frequency. For all procedures in our blood bank in an 18 month period, there were 195 errors of identification, 842 errors of transcription, etc. (Table II) for a total of almost 2500 errors, what seems at first to be an outrageously large number of errors. If examined in terms of functions, however, there were only 195 errors of identification out of 7.5 million times (Table III) that our personnel identified a patient or unit of blood. An error rate of only 0.003% is almost more than can be expected from human beings!

If these error rates are rounded off, they fall into three general groups (Table IV). Errors of storage and retrieval (key entry errors not accepted by the computer) occur approximately 1 in every 1000 times that information is stored or retrieved in a

Table IV. Blood bank errors: Approximate frequency.

	By Function	By Procedure
Storage & retrieval	1/1000	1/100
Identification, performance, transcription	1/10,000	1/1000
Interpretation	1/100,000	1/10,000

computer system. For the functions of identification, performance and transcription, the error rate is approximately 1 in 10,000 times that function is performed. Errors of interpretation occur extremely rarely, approximately 1 per 100,000. Although, these functional error rates are extremely low, it must be remembered that for each procedure, each function may be performed numerous times i.e., in the ABO/Rh typing procedure there are 4 steps of interpretation, 7 transcription steps, etc. Nevertheless, if only one transcription error is made, an incorrect ABO type may be reported. As a result, it is no longer important that a transcription error occurs only 1 in 10,000 transcriptions; more important is the frequency with which the final product of the entire procedure will be in error. When we examined our error rates, not in terms of function, but, as others have done, in terms of the final product, the procedural error rate (Table IV) was observed to be much higher (by a multiple of approximately 10). These unacceptably high procedural or final product error rates of 1/100 to 1/1000 which we and others have observed in retrospective studies, have mislead us, in the past, to introduce numerous checks and double-checks into our procedures and to exhort our laboratory personnel to improve unacceptable performance in terms of end product, they really reflect very good performance in terms of function. Through prospective error analysis, we have recognized that procedural error rates (or an error in the final product) as high as 1/100, can result from functional error rates as low as 1/10,000. Since it is not reasonable to expect human error to occur with a frequency of less than 1/10,000, the only way to improve the procedural error rate, (i.e., the final product error rate) is by making major system changes. It is not sufficiently safe to rely on people to transcribe information from one piece of paper to another or to rely on people to file an ABO/Rh report slip in the right location in a file cabinet without making errors with unacceptable frequency. Only with major system changes, such as the use of a computer file, can we significantly change error rates and have reliable storage and retrieval of ABO/Rh types.

ERROR CONTROL BY SYSTEM CHANGE

Our most common errors were those of storage and retrieval of vital patient information, i.e., ABO/Rh type, presence of an irregular antibody and transfusion precautions and instructions. In some emergency situations, rapid retrieval of information of this type could be critical for that patient's life. In our initial study (9), we found that over a period of about 3 years, 2 to 3 out of every 100 reports filed could no longer be found. Of the 7256 functional errors detected in our blood bank at this time, one of the most commen (40%), was filing error. With implementation of a computer file for storage and retrieval of patient information, our error rate (10) dropped from 2.6% to 0.25% (Fig. 6). In fact, our procedural error rate with the computer system is 0. The 0.25% error rate reflects only functional or key entry errors which are not accepted by the computer.

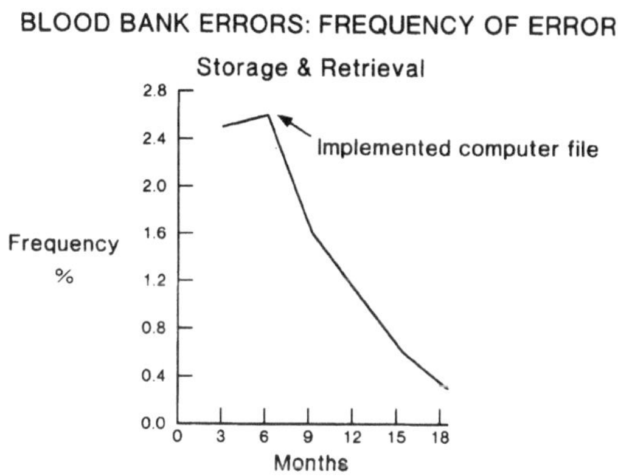

Figure 6.

ERROR FREQUENCY: BY ACTIVITY AND OVERALL

It is also informative to analyze error frequency after categorizing errors into one of the three general locations or types of blood bank activities. 1) Collection and processing activities which take place in donor collection centers include preparation of donor materials, phlebotomy, ABO/Rh type, etc. 2) Compatibility testing within the hospital laboratory includes ABO/Rh type, antibody screen and the crossmatch. 3) The administration or transfusion of blood which in most institutions is done by the hospital medical or nursing staff (and not by the blood bank at all). At our institution, since we in the blood bank are responsible for all three types of activity, we have had an opportunity to observe and analyze the frequency and types of errors in all three of these blood bank and transfusion activities. When 2498 errors observed in our blood bank over an 18 month period were categorized by activity (Table V), the largest number, almost 1200, occurred in the compatibility testing laboratory; the smalles number, 413 occurred in the process of administering blood; and an intermediate number, 904, occurred during collection and processing. However,

Table V. Blood bank errors: By Activity (in 18 months)

Activity	Number of Errors
Collection and processing	904
Compatibility	1181
Administration	413
Total	2498

Table VI. Blood bank errors: By activity and frequency of function (in 18 months).

	%	
Collection and processing	0.007	$= \frac{904}{12,213,981}$
Compatibility	0.012	$= \frac{1181}{9,600,000}$
Administration	0.008	$= \frac{413}{5,488,931}$

Numerator: Sum of all errors within activity.
Denominator: Sum of frequency of all functions.

Table VII. Blood bank errors: By activity and frequency of final product (in 18 months).

	%	
Collection and processing	1.5	$= \frac{904}{60,205}$
Compatibility	0.08	$= \frac{1181}{157,921}$
Administration	1.2	$= \frac{413}{35,765}$

Numerator: Sum of all errors within activity.
Denominator: Number of units collected, crossmatched or transfused.

when these three quite different numbers are divided by their functional activity denominators (Table VI), it becomes apparent that the functional error rates in all three types of activity in the Mayo Clinic Blood Bank and Transfusion Service are very similar, 0.007 to 0.012 or approximately 1/10,000. While a functional error rate of only 1/10,000 may seem acceptable, this low error rate, nevertheless gives rise to a final product error rate (Table VII) in each area of approximately 1/100! Fortunately, many of these errors are trivial and usually (but not always) do not result in significant morbidity or mortality. A reduction in this error rate, however, will not occur until major changes are made in our systems for transcription, identification, performance, etc.

An error reporting and analysis system also permits observation of the overall error rate in the blood bank over a period of time. A major change in overall error rate (Fig. 7) occurred in our blood bank during 1979 as a result of the introduction of a computer for storage and retrieval of patient information. Our overall procedural error rate dropped from approximately 0.17 to 0.05 and remained stable throughout 1980. In 1981, our error rate abruptly began to rise. Since we had recently hired many new nurses and clerks, we analyzed the error rate for a specific procedure, the blood donor phlebotomy, since it would reflect nursing and clerical personnel changes more dramatically than the overall blood bank error rate. When error rates for the donor

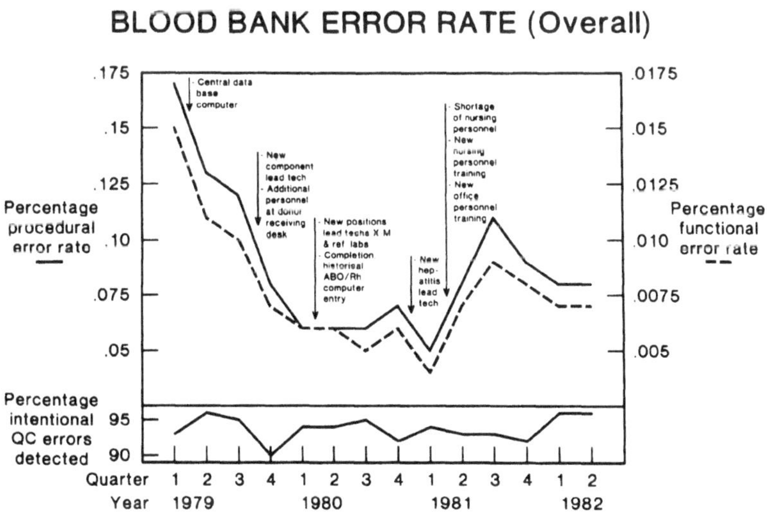

Figure 7.

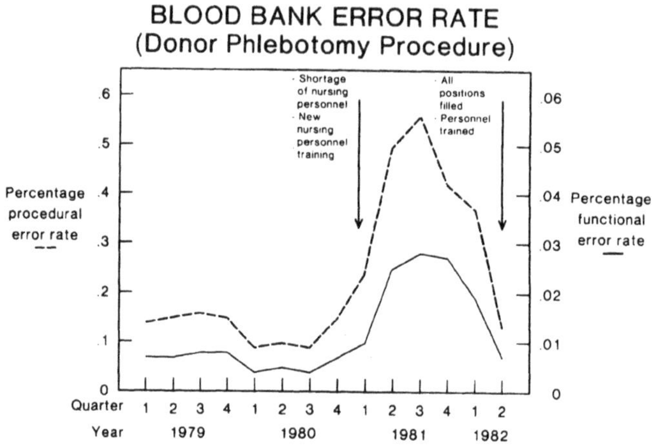

Figure 8.

phlebotomy procedure were calculated and graphed (Fig. 8), an increase could be noted by the end of 1980 with a dramatic rise occurring during 1981, and a gradual decline by the end of 1981 to baseline levels in mid 1982. This rise and decline in error rates for the donor phlebotomy procedure coincided with the large turnover in our nurse phlebotomists and clerical personnel and the gradual replacement and training of new personnel.

CONCLUSIONS

A new functional classification of errors has been developed which permits categorization of all blood bank errors into one of five functions: identification, performance, transcription, interpretation and storage and retrieval. When combined with a system for identification and reporting of all blood bank errors, it becomes possible to determine error frequency by function, by procedure and by location or type of activity. Armed with information of this type, it is possible to compare error rates over a period of time; after appropriate corrective action; and after changes in reagents, equipment, procedures or personnel. Use of this system in our blood bank has made apparent to us that even minimal functional error rates can produce unacceptably high procedural or end product error rates which can be reduced only by major system changes. Finally, this system of error reporting and analysis provides a mechanism with which to compare performance between blood banks and to establish minimum standards of performance.

REFERENCES

1. Schmidt, P.J., Kevy, S.V. Sources of Error in a Hospital Blood Bank. Transfusion 1963;3:198–201.
2. Kwa, S.B., Ariff, K.B. Blood Banking Errors: A Two Year Prospective Survey. Singapore Med. J. 1966;7:178–84.
3. Lacerte, J.M., Kane, V.M., Cohen, P. U.S. Licensed Blood Banks: Evaluation of Whole Blood and Its Components. Transfusion 1972;12:339–43.
4. Taswell, H.F., Smith, A.M., Sweatt, M.A., Pfaff, K.J. Quality Control in the Blood Bank — A new Approach. American Journal of Clinical Pathology 1974;62:491–5.
5. Schmidt, P.J. Transfusion Mortality: With Special Reference to Surgical and Intensive Care Facilities. J. Fla. Med. Assn. 1980;67:151–3.
6. Schmidt, P.J. The Mortality from Incompatible Transfusion. In: Progress in Clinical and Biological Research, Vol. 43, Sandler, S.G., Nusbacher, J., Schanfield, M.S. eds., Alan R. Liss, Inc., 1980:251–61.
7. Honig, C.L., Bove, J.R. Transfusion Associated Fatalities: Review of Bureau of Biologics Reports 1976–1878. Transfusion 1980;20:653–61.
8. Myhre, B. Fatalities from Blood Transfusion. JAMA 1980;244: 1333–5.
9. Taswell, H.F., Sonnenberg, C.L. Blood Bank Errors: A New Functional Classification. Transfusion 1979;19:652–3 (abstract).
10. Taswell, H.F., Sonnenberg, C.L. Blood Bank Errors: Classification and Frequency. Transfusion 1982;21:620–1 (abstract).

ERROR ANALYSIS: METHODS OF DETECTION, ANALYSIS AND CONTROL

C.L. Sonnenberg, H.F. Taswell

Significant transfusion morbidity and mortality result from human error (1,2,3). To minimize errors, it is necessary to acquire knowledge of these errors and their frequency by 1) monitoring for, collecting and analyzing actual errors, and 2) introducing intentional errors and following their course through the system.

There are five objectives in the actual error program: 1) to collect information about various types of errors and the rate at which these errors occur, 2) to recognize systems or procedures that are prone to error, 3) to monitor personnel using the established systems and procedures, 4) to introduce specific changes to prevent reoccurrence of errors, and 5) once changes have been made, to monitor the effect of these changes on personnel, systems and procedures.

To collect information in an actual error program, personnel are asked to record all errors on an Error Report Form (Figure 1). This form provides a record of the date, patient or donor identification information, a brief description of the error, the location in which the error originated i.e. crossmatch laboratory, donor physical examination area, or clerical area, and the location in which the error was found.

Date	Patient I.D.	Description of Error	Area Originated	Area Found

Figure 1. Error Report Form.

To analyze the error in more detail, an Error Analysis Report (Figure 2) has been developed which requests: the name of the person completing the report, the date and time the error occurred, whether it occurred in a routine or emergency situation, the names of all personnel involved, a more detailed description of the error and recommendations for changes in methods or per-

Name of person making report ______________________________

Date/time of error ____________ Routine ______ Emergency ___

Personnel Involved (blood bank, nurse, MD, patient, etc. _____

____

Description of Error ______________________________________

____

Has the error been reviewed with the person involved? _ Yes _ No

To avoid recurrence of this type of error, the following changes should be made in:

a. Methods ______________________________________

b. Personnel ____________________________________

Figure 2. Error Analysis Report.

sonnel. It is important that the person(s) responsible for an error are informed of the error and, in fact, may be the best person to describe the error and suggest any changes that may be necessary. Collecting actual errors in this manner permits a blood bank: 1) to evaluate error rates, and 2) to categorize errors by function. As a result, all errors can be classified into five functions; identification, performance, interpretation, transcription and storage and retrieval.

To categorize errors by function, it is first necessary to identify all technical and administrative blood bank procedures critical for patient safety (e.g. ABO/Rh typing, labeling and administration of blood products etc.). Each step in each of these procedures must then be categorized by function and the frequency of each function determined for the procedure.

These steps can be illustrated (Figure 3) using the ABO/Rh Typing Procedure as an example. 1) This procedure usually begins with a comparison of the identification labels on the blood sample and on the transfusion request form. This function is one of <u>identification</u> and since it is performed once by the venipuncturist, <u>the frequency</u> of this function is one in this step, but six for the entire ABO/Rh typing procedure. 2) Once identification has been assured, it is generally necessary to transfer the identification information from the request form onto the ABO/Rh Report form. This is a function of <u>transcription</u> and its frequency is one in this step and seven in <u>this procedure</u>. 3) After a blood sample has been collected, a 2% red cell suspension must be prepared. This function is categorized as <u>performance</u> and its frequency is one in this step and 11 for the <u>entire procedure</u>. 4) Subsequently, when results of serum and cell typing are available, they must be interpreted. This is a function of <u>interpretation</u> with a frequency of four since two different <u>technologists</u> each independently

Function	Frequency (factor)
Identification	6
1. Compare sample and report form x1	
Performance	11
1. Prepare 2% patient RBC suspension x1	
7. Add 1 drop anti-A to tube x1	
Interpretation	4
1. Interpret ABO serum typing x1	
2. Interpret ABO cell typing x1	
3. Interpret Rho(D) typing x2	
Transcription	7
1. Transfer ID from request to report x1	
4. Record results on report form x4	
Storage and Retrieval	2
1. Enter results in computer x2	

Figure 3. Error Analysis: Methods.
Example: Worksheet for Error Categorization ABO/Rh Typing.

interpret ABO serum or cell plus Rh type. 5) Finally, the report is filed for future reference. This is a function of storage and retrieval and the frequency is two for the procedure.

After each step in a procedure has been categorized by function and frequency, the entire procedure can be described in terms of each function and its frequency. In our example of ABO typing, as performed in our blood bank, there are six steps of identification, seven of transcription, eleven of performance, four of interpretation and two of storage and retrieval. The frequency (or function factor) of each of these functions is subsequently used to calculate error rates using the formulas shown in Figure 4. Error rates should be calculated periodically (monthly, at our blood bank) for each of the five functions as well as the overall Procedural and Functional Error Rates for the entire blood bank or selected areas within the blood bank.

$$\%\ \text{Procedural Error Rate} = \frac{\text{Number of Errors}}{\text{Number of Procedures}} \times 100$$

$$\%\ \text{Functional Error Rate} = \frac{\text{Number of Errors}}{\text{Number of Procedures} \times \text{Function Factor*}} \times 100$$

* Function Factor = Number of steps of a particular function in the procedure.

Figure 4. Error Rate: Formulas

The following briefly described situations are two examples of the types of errors that may be reported in your blood bank and will be used for illustrative purposes.

1. The current ABO type of a patient was found to be type A, however when compared with an historical type, it was noted that the patient was previously type 0. The ABO type was repeated on a current blood sample, and confirmed to be type 0. Upon further investigation, it was found that the technician had used another patient's blood sample for ABO typing.
2. In another, more common error, a clerk transcribed the donor identification number incorrectly onto the laboratory report.

The error in the first example should be classified as an identification error. In the hypothetical example (Figure 5), one identification error was found during a time period in which 1000 ABO/Rh typings were performed yielding a procedural error rate of 0.1%. If the number of procedures performed (1000) is multiplied by the number of identification steps (6), it is apparent that the total number of identification steps performed during the time period was 6000 and, therefore, that the functional error rate for steps of identification was 0.017%.

Procedure	No. of Errors	Factor	No. of Proc.	Factor x Proc.	% Proc. Error Rate	% Funct. Error Rate
ABO/Rh Typing	1	6	1000	6000	0.10	0.017
Donor Material Preparation	1	10	5000	50000	0.02	0.002

Figure 5. Calculation of Error Rates: Examples of Identification and Transcription.

The error in the second example should be classified as a transcription error. In this case (Figure 5), one transcription error was found when preparing donor materials for 5000 donors, a procedural error rate of 0.02%. If the number of procedures performed (5000) is multiplied by the number of transcription steps (10), the total number of transcription steps performed during the time period measured was 50,000 or a functional error rate of 0.002%.

Once procedural and functional error rates have been calculated for each procedure or function, these rates can be graphed versus time. If error rates are observed to increase significantly over a period of time, necessary changes in personnel, systems or procedures can be initiated and then the effect can be monitored by again observing the error rates over a subsequent period of time.

Reliable identification and reporting of actual errors is vital for accurate calculation of error rates. The success of the actual error program and the validity of its results is entirely dependent on the support and cooperation of both the personnel and management of the blood bank. To measure this support and the reliability of actual error detection and reporting, it is necessary to introduce an intentional error program (4,5) as a system of control for the actual error program.

There are two objectives of an intentional error program: 1) To measure the detection rate of intentional errors which then permits calculation of a corrected detection rate for actual errors, and 2) to raise the level of awareness of personnel to specific types of errors.

If intentional errors reflect the type of errors which are actually occurring, then, the detection rate of intentional errors should provide a measure of the rate of detection of actual errors as well as a measure of the attitude of personnel to the error control program. Intentional errors should also be selected for each type of actual error by function. Several examples follow:

1) To reproduce an intentional error of identification a blood sample could be labeled with incorrect identification information. The technician using that blood sample should recognize this error when performing the identification step in the test procedure.

2) A measure of one type of performance error can be obtained by sending the laboratory technician a serum sample with a weak (but detectable) red blood cell antibody. This example will measure the competency of personnel and whether their performance conforms with the standard procedure.

3) One type of interpretation error can be evaluated through use of a blood sample which has been modified to be read as an ABO mixed field if properly interpreted.

4) Detection of transcription errors could be evaluated by intentionally entering a donor identification number incorrectly on one of the many donor processing forms which must be checked by various individuals during the donation process.

5) Storage and retrieval error detection was evaluated in our laboratory (prior to development of our computer system) by intentionally misfiling a report to determine if the clerk responsible for double-checking the filing of the report would recognize the error.

The example of an intentional transcription error cited above is identical with the second hypothetical actual error previously described. The transcription error whether actual or intentional should be recognized by the donor physical examination nurse whose responsibility it is to recheck all donor processing materials for accuracy. The percent failure to detect an intentional error of transcription will therefore provide a measure of the rate of detection of actual transcription errors.

It is important to consider who will perform and coordinate day-to-day tasks of error control. It is essential to develop a quality control technologist position with defined responsibilities. The size of the laboratory will dictate whether the amount of time needed to fulfill these responsibilities would require a full-time or part-time position. The individual selected for this position should have 1) a thorough understanding of all systems and procedures within the blood bank, and 2) be able to communicate and work well with others. Support and input from both management and employees are essential for a successful program which can only be achieved with positive attitudes toward the program. It must be made clear to personnel that this program is not intended to find fault with any individual but, to gain information that can be used to improve patient services.

One of the primary responsibilities of the quality control technologist is to develop and write procedures for the initiation, follow-up and data collection of intentional errors. We have found that the "Playscript" procedure (6), often called the "Responsibility/Action" procedure format (7), works well for these procedures. For example (Figure 6), clerical personnel, in collaboration with the quality control technologist, should periodically purposely initiate an error such as intentionally recording an incorrect donor identification number on the laboratory report form or other donor processing materials. This intentional error should be detected by the physical examination nurse. If the error is detected, the nurse will report the error to the clerical personnel. The error would then be allowed to continue on in the system to the donor phlebotomy nurse who should detect the error and would then, again, report it to the clerical personnel. If the error is not detected by either nurse, it is the responsibility of clerical personnel to follow that error, correct it and record on the worksheet that the error was not recognized by either nurse.

Responsibility	Action
Clerical Personnel	Purposely initiate error
Physical Exam Nurse Phlebotomy Nurse	Expect detection
Clerical Personnel	Responsible for follow-up if error not detected by nurse

Figure 6. Intentional Error: Playscript Procedure.

It is essential to develop worksheets of this type (Figure 7) for the collection of data on intentional errors, as well as to ensure that there is follow-up so that the error is corrected if it has not been detected by personnel. The worksheet should include: 1) the date, 2) the correct donor identification number, 3) a description of the error, and 4) columns to record whether personnel detected or missed the intentional error. It is important for the quality control technologist to monitor the intentional error pro-

Date	Donor ID	Description of Error	PE Area		Phlebotomy Area	
			Detected	Missed	Detected	Missed

Figure 7. Intentional Errors: Worksheet.
Example: Clerical Checks – Donor Material.

gram to ensure that procedures are being followed and problems being addressed and resolved on a timely basis. The intentional error data must be collected throughout the blood bank and analyzed by the quality control technologist on a periodic basis. Detection rates can then be calculated by dividing the number of errors detected by the number of errors initiated and multiplying by 100. Analysis of the data and calculation of detection rates can be looked at from the standpoint of 1) work area, i.e., clerical, crossmatch or donor collection area, 2) by function, i.e., identification, transcription, performance, etc., or 3) by procedure, i.e., ABO/Rh typing, donor processing materials preparation, etc. These detection rates provide an on-going measure of how well personnel are recognizing and reporting errors seeded into the system and therefore, a measure of the detection rate of actual errors. When the intentional error program was first implemented in our blood bank, detection rates were less than 50% but rapidly increased and have remained in the range of 95% for many years. Thus, 95% of actual errors are probably being recognized in our blood bank and the percent procedural and functional error rates can be corrected for the percent of errors not recognized. Both actual and intentional error detection rates should be graphed versus time; the latter serving as a control for the former. Appropriate corrective action should be taken if 1) the rate of detection of intentional errors falls, or 2) the rate of detection of actual errors increases significantly. After corrective action has been taken, error rates should be observed for improvement.

In summary, errors in a blood bank and transfusion service must be identified and categorized, their frequency determined and followed periodically with appropriate corrective changes introduced and the effects of these changes monitored if we are to reach the goal of safe and effective transfusion.

REFERENCES

1. Honig, C.L., Bove, J.R. Transfusion Associated Fatalities: Review of Bureau of Biologics Reports 1976–1978, Transfusion 1980;20:653–61.

2. Myhre, B. Fatalities From Blood Transfusion. JAMA 1980;244: 1333–5.
3. Schmidt, P. The Mortality From Incompatible Transfusion. In: Progress in Clinical and Biological Research, Vol. 43, Sandler, S.G., Nusbacher, J., Schanfield, M.S. (eds.) Alan R. Liss, Inc., pp. 251–61.
4. Taswell, H.F., et al. Quality Control in the Blood Bank — A New Approach. Am. J. Clin. Pathol. 1974;62:491–5.
5. Taswell, H.F. Error Production and Its Control. In: A Seminar on Performance Evaluation, American Association of Blood Banks Publication 1976:115–20.
6. The Playscript Procedure. A New Tool of Administration, Leslie, H. Matthies, Office Publications, Inc., New York, 1961.
7. Beattie, K.M., Hanson, M., Taswell, H.F. Systems and Procedures. In: Taswell, H.F., Saeed, S.M. (eds.) Principles and Practice of Quality Control in the Blood Bank. American Association of Blood Banks Publication, 1980:121–2.

DISCUSSION

Moderators: R.E. Klein, C.Th. Smit Sibinga

P.J. Schmidt, Tampa, USA:

I certainly would like to congratulate the speakers on this analysis. As I remember the paper by Lacerte*, the label error rate was one to every three, on donor blood products inspected by the Division of Biological Standards, now the FDA. The inspector goes to a regional centre, takes a sample product and sends it in to main headquarters in Washington. The fact that they were finding one in three products to be falsely labeled, seems to me a perfect illustration of what Dr. Högman described as looking under the street light when the key was dropped "over there". They were reporting "errors" of no significance which were violations of insignificant rules and regulations. When rules and regulations are so silly, that one time out of three somebody cannot follow them, they need to be changed.

C.F. Högman, Uppsala, Sweden:

I also enjoyed this presentation. But what I would like to ask is the apparent fact that the errors may have different values. Some of them may be very dangerous, others may have less importance. I think that in any well-functioning organization, a certain security system has been built up in such a way that if an error occurs somewhere, there should be a possibility to detect it. It is very common to repeat testings and do this separately in order to be able to detect mistakes. In my own experience, I have found that it is surprising how many controls are needed before you actually detect the error. I wonder if you have any comment on that?

Another thing which I would like to emphasize – which Dr. Taswell has shown so intelligently – is that the introduction of computers in our routine activity can actually make the whole procedure much safer. The nice thing about computers is that they have such a big memory. You can store data for hundreds of thousands of patients, which could be very quickly checked, if you have a repeat test. In my own institution, we have our own computer which is operated on a 24-hour basis and which is used

* Lacerte, J.M. et al. Transfusion 1972;12:339–43.

for printing out replies about blood type and other serological information. This is used in the cross-matching laboratory, and also for checking the historical data. In this way, we feel we have a means to prevent mistakes on the part of the laboratory.

H.F. Taswell:

I believe that any error one makes is an important error. Clearly if, you walk up to the wrong patient and transfuse him with a unit of blood, that is a pretty important error. But are there also unimportant errors? I do not believe that anymore and if there are unimportant errors, there are very few. Let me give you an example of an "unimportant" error. Suppose you received a patient's blood sample for cross-matching, and a transfusion request card with the spelling of the patient's name differing slightly between blood sample and request card. This is obviously a "trivial" mistake which we can ignore. The only problem is, that there are two patients each with names spelled slightly differently. Serious reaction is the result.

In another situation: One patient's name was "John Doe" and the other was "John Doe Jr.". Unimportant mistake? Not worth bothering with? However, one happened to be the father who was donating a kidney to the son. The wrong person got the blood. I really do not think there is a mistake which is unimportant.

One last comment. There is a book, which was written a number of years ago, I think it was called "Collision Course". It was the true story of the sinking of a major steamship. The whole gist of that book was how a whole series of very "trivial" and "unimportant" mistakes all came together and sank a ship*.

C.F. Högman:

I tend to disagree somewhat. I thought you took a very bad example, since identification has always been one of the most important areas. The example you gave illustrates how careful you have to be in order to perform the correct identification. I could also give examples about confusion in names. What this tells us is that we really have to have a system of identification which is unique for the patient. In our country, there is such a system, based on numbers. In the Blood Transfusion Services, this is extremely useful. However, it could be questioned from the point of view of "Big Brother".

R.J. Crawford, Glasgow, Scotland:

The point I really want to make to Dr. Taswell is in connection with trivial errors. We have been told by some of our staff that if a mistake is made and is immediately detected within the oper-

* Moscow, A. Collision Course. London, Longman, Brill & Co., 1959.

ating systems of the particular procedure which is being carried out, then it should not be reportable as an error, because it has already been detected by the operating system. If one accidentally puts a drop of reagent in the wrong tube, pulls the tube out and throws it away and replaces it with the correct tube, is this the kind of error you would audit?

H.F. Taswell:

I am glad you brought that up. We have a number of years ago in a publication*, made a distinction between what we defined as "errors" and "discrepancies". By definition, an error is a mistake made, which leaves your Blood Bank and is discovered by someone outside of the Blood Bank. A discrepancy is a mistake, which someone catches, and it never leaves the Blood Bank, because your system worked, and caught it. We are not talking about discrepancies, we are talking about errors. Not trivial errors, but errors that escaped us – real errors – that the system did not catch. I guess I would have to disagree with Dr. Högman. People make mistakes in funny ways, and you do not learn it until you start looking at 2,500 mistakes.

Ch.A. Schiffer, Baltimore, USA:

I think the next extension, and maybe the next publication will have to deal with how much it costs to correct and constantly catch errors of different types. This is the overwhelming reality we are all being crushed by, because there are obviously errors of varying magnitude, most of which probably do not make their way to the bed-side in terms of clinical importance. The computer is probably a cheap way of correcting some of the errors, because it replaces personnel. But, there are lots of other errors for which repetitive testing is done which probably might not stand cost-effective scrutiny.

H.F. Taswell:

We are very aware of the question of cost-effectiveness. We cannot evaluate that, yet, except in a very limited way, because what we are doing now is research, not routine service. We could evaluate cost-effectiveness, however, on services that we have implemented, like the use of a computer for storage and retrieval of ABO typing information. This is a system that is running, it is not research. In looking at our costs for the storage and retrieval of ABO typing information, it is very cost-effective. It is much cheaper now – even forgetting the errors that are eliminated – than it was before. But, I agree that it is very important that with any method that is introduced, you must look at what the cost is and see what you are getting for it.

* Taswell, H.F. In: A seminar on performance evaluation. Chicago, Ill., Gunthorp-Warren Printing Co., 1976, pp. 115–20

I would like to make one or two other comments. One is something I referred to at the end of my talk when I said that this system provides a basis for establishing standards of performance with regard to error control. I think this is one area of quality control which has not been mentioned and is somewhere in the future evolution of blood banking from art to science. We must establish certain minimum standards of performance. As an example, a certain error rate is considered acceptable, or a certain measure of the quality of a blood donor pool is considered acceptable or unacceptable. This is a very difficult, but important area which we will have to develop over the years ahead.

Lastly, I would like to complement Dr. Smit Sibinga and all his co-workers for a really excellent symposium and for all the time, attention and care that they put into producing this symposium – with virtually no error.

GPSR Compliance
The European Union's (EU) General Product Safety Regulation (GPSR) is a set of rules that requires consumer products to be safe and our obligations to ensure this.

If you have any concerns about our products, you can contact us on

ProductSafety@springernature.com

In case Publisher is established outside the EU, the EU authorized representative is:

Springer Nature Customer Service Center GmbH
Europaplatz 3
69115 Heidelberg, Germany

www.ingramcontent.com/pod-product-compliance
Ingram Content Group UK Ltd.
Pitfield, Milton Keynes, MK11 3LW, UK
UKHW020801290926
15470UKWH00003B/878
* 9 7 8 0 8 9 8 3 8 6 1 8 9 *